The Paty Plan

Seth -
To success in L.A. and to a happy,
healthy life!

Katharine E. Paty

The Paty Plan

Flavor Without Fat
An eight-week guide to permanent
weight loss

Katharine Edmonds Paty

VANTAGE PRESS
New York

The recipes herein have not been tested by the publisher.

Cover Designer: Ann Williamson
Cover Illustrator: Ann Williamson

FIRST EDITION

Published by Vantage Press, Inc.
516 West 34th Street, New York, New York 10001

Manufactured in the United States of America
ISBN: 0-533-14044-7

Library of Congress Catalog Card No.: 01-126837

0 9 8 7 6 5 4 3 2 1

To the slimmer love of my life, Art, who graciously endured all of my low-fat culinary successes and failures.

Contents

Author's Note

This "diet" is not based on scientific evidence. Consult your physi-
cian before you commence with this or any other weight loss plan.

Acknowledgments

Special thanks to:

All the wonderful chefs in the world whose inspiration helped me create many of the recipes in this book.

Janet Edmonds for showing her faith in extraordinary ways.

Philippa Kingsley-Perel and Margaret C. Price who tried to surround me with the "right people."

Ben Edmonds and Kathy Cromartie who lent their editing expertise and so much more.

Barbara Rubin who interpreted my handwritten hieroglyphics and moved me into the computer age.

Kathleen Zelman whose knowledge of nutrition has been invaluable.

Ann Williamson for her boundless creativity.

Vantage Press, Inc. for turning my dream into a visual reality.

Janet and Benjamin Edmonds, Ann Williamson, Sally Kellogg, Rigby Barnes, Betty Hanson, Deke Grinnell and Bill Summerour: you are the ones who encouraged me all the way.

Harvie and Chuck Abney for making *The Paty Plan* their plan for life.

Foreword

Review of Katharine Paty's Low-fat Cookbook
By Kathleen Zelman, M.P.H., R.D.
June 15, 2001

Eating nutritiously is an essential part of good health along with a lifestyle that includes regular physical exercise. In our society, the average American consumes too many calories and too much fat in their diet. This lifestyle, coupled with too little exercise, has resulted in skyrocketing numbers of overweight and obese people. In order to lose weight and reduce the risk of chronic disease, most of us need to focus on a healthier lifestyle, which includes a low-fat, low-calorie diet and a firm commitment to daily activity.

Katharine Paty's book, *The Paty Plan*, is just what the doctor ordered. Katharine has clearly demonstrated that low-fat and healthy cuisine is easy to prepare and, above all, delicious. Her innovative approach to enhancing flavor without added fat will enlighten cooks and delight everyone who enjoys her recipes. The collection of recipes is simple, easy and fun. Cooks will learn her tricks and techniques to lower the fat content without sacrificing flavor. These tempting and enjoyable recipes will satisfy the most discriminating palates.

The majority of ingredients in the recipes come from nature's bounty and form the base of the USDA Food Guide Pyramid. These nutritious foods are the foundation of a diet rich in vitamins, minerals and fiber and are chock full of phytochemicals, nutrients that protect against disease. In addition, most of the foods are naturally fat-free. The majority of the recipes are vegetarian and thus contain trace amounts of fat. Recipes that include poultry, seafood or canned soup yield a maximum of ten grams of fat per serving. The only exceptions are the salmon recipes which are slightly higher in fat (nine grams of fat per three-ounce cooked portion), however, this type of fat contains omega-3 fatty acids which offer wonderful health benefits.

Katharine's passion and knowledge of food comes together in this cookbook and is a real treat for anyone who is interested in healthy cuisine that is simply delicious. Bon Appetit!

—Kathleen Zelman, M.P.H., R.D.

A Letter to the Reader

Dear Reader,

It is a privilege to write in praise of Katharine Paty and *THE PATY PLAN*. After gaining weight over a five-year period, I tried all the standard ways to lose the extra pounds—meetings, weight-loss programs, exercise at the gym and with a personal trainer. My success was minimal. Very discouraged and feeling unhappy over my appearance, I heard from Katharine (my caterer for parties) of her *PATY PLAN*. It is my salvation, and my husband Chuck has suggested we build a shrine in honor of her "miraculous work!"

I've lost a considerable number of pounds since beginning the program. Every week that I have eaten according to plan, I have lost a minimum of two pounds, and some weeks the scales register a loss of three or four pounds! This is so encouraging to me. I see results.

The good news does not end there. The food on the plan is absolutely delicious and filling. I never feel denied and there are no bland flavors in the recipes. Katharine has done something marvelous with seasonings and herbs. Black Beans with Rice, Turkey Taco Ensalada and her Tomato Aspic top my list of favorite recipes. My husband adores her Fish and Corn Creole and her Seafood Pita Sandwich.

The greatest testament I can give Katharine is that, except for an occasional Crème Brûlée, I intend to follow her directions for life. I encourage others to do the same.

Sincerely,

Harvie Abney

Introduction

My fortieth year loomed heavily over my horizon. Sadly, "heavy" became the adjective that increasingly displayed itself in the beachside birthday celebration photographs. All my aspirations to be a svelte mid-lifer vanished as I viewed the video and photo documentation that immortalized the big event.

Another seven months passed and a few more pounds were gained. Enough was enough! The year was 1995. Oprah was talking low-fat with Rosie. Dr. Art Ulene said to count the fat grams. Reducing the fat intake in my diet seemed like a sensible, healthy way to shed unwanted pounds. But how do I go about losing the weight? What do I eat on a day-to-day basis? If I take the weight off, how do I keep it off?

The questions did not end there. As owner of Festivities, Inc., an Atlanta-based party planning consultant firm, the taste and presentation of food is paramount to me. Cooking is my passion and eating the number one love of my husband's life. (I rank number two!) Therefore my challenge became multifaceted. How do I go about losing weight and counting fat grams while satisfying both my culinary yearnings and my husband's taste buds?

In search of the answer to my first two questions, I browsed through bookstores looking for a "low-fat diet" that would tell me what to eat each day. Failing to find one, I decided to design my own program. I read that one would lose weight by keeping fat grams to ten-twenty per day. The grocery store became my research library. With current nutritional labels, counting fat grams has never been easier. My findings confirmed what my heart already knew. Vegetables are golden. Red meat, cheese, butter and poultry skin are the villains. Energy-boosting, carbohydrate-rich pasta and breads would incorporate themselves beautifully into what was to become a lifetime eating plan. While having no educational training in nutrition, it seemed to me that this new dietary approach would also be low in cholesterol. What a wonderful added benefit.

I began my diet on April 29, 1995. My husband Art and I were being entertained lavishly at a cocktail party. I decided not to partake of any of the tempting hors d'oeuvres. Going out to dinner afterwards, I ordered a salad with balsamic vinegar. I had turned a corner. By the time of my stepdaughter's July 8, 1995 wedding, I had lost fifteen pounds. Another five disappeared by Labor Day. During the Christmas season, I was celebrating the loss of thirty pounds and my husband was celebrating his weight loss with me!

In this book I am going to share with you how we lost our excess baggage. The "do's" and "don'ts" of our diet will be in the first section. I will then guide you through an eight-week plan unraveling the mystery of what to eat each day. Lastly, you will find the low-fat recipes I created or adapted, not only for weight loss, but to satisfy the gourmet in me and the gourmand in my husband. They are recipes we prepare today to maintain our slimmer figures and our new healthier lifestyle.

While my family will attest to the fact that I am no athlete, this book would not be complete without a word on exercise. No healthy lifestyle plan will work without it. I considered myself physically dormant in April of 1995. I now try to power walk three miles four times a week. My goal is to exceed that and to be as consistent with my exercise routine as I am with my eating habits.

Finally, it is important to remember that this book is not just about losing weight. It is about not starving yourself in order to obtain a slimmer waistline. It is about developing and maintaining beneficial eating habits. It is about flavor without fat. It is about celebrating food that is not only good for you but delectable to the palate.

I now extend all my best to you as you travel the road to a slimmer, healthier and more energetic you. Good luck!

The Paty Plan

The Do's and the Don'ts of The Paty Plan

While I was putting my low-fat plan on paper and experimenting with recipes, a friend of my mother's asked if she could have butter on my diet. She was also curious to know if meals prepared with low-fat ingredients tasted the same as ones comprised of foods high in fat. The answers to both inquiries was no. But believe it or not, it did not take me long to discover that I personally relished a butterless, salted and peppered baked potato. I learned that delicacies like asparagus need no enhancement. Sliced turkey breast with cranberry sauce took on an elevated status at my dinner table. The low-fat taste I initially experienced evaporated. Good taste became synonymous with the bountiful foods found in the world's gardens and oceans. I hope you experience similar awakenings as you embark upon the following dietary plan.

Another question was asked by my fried chicken, potato chip eating friend. She wanted to know if she would have plenty to eat during the weight-reducing phase of my program. I assured her that there is no need to count calories or place puny poultry pieces on scales. Do not even be obsessed with how many fat grams are in your plump grilled chicken breast. Just make sure it is skinless. Identifying and consuming low-fat foods in moderate quantities is the key to success. Eating sensibly is about moderation, not deprivation.

All your pertinent questions should be answered when you become acquainted with the following list of "do's" and "don'ts." I think you will be pleasantly surprised to learn that the guidelines are simple. Just familiarize yourself with the fat gram information on food package labeling and the rest of the rules are easy. To discover just how easy, turn the page and the essence of *The Paty Plan* will be revealed.

Life is not fair. In order to lose weight, women need to keep their fat intake closer to ten grams. Most men can get away with consuming almost twice that amount while watching the needle on the scales descend. Each individual will need to determine what works best.

Do

1. Read fat gram labels.
2. Keep daily fat grams below 20. (My optimum weight loss occurred when I consumed around 10 per day. Remember, the lower the fat grams, the greater the weight loss.)
3. Remove all skin from chicken and fish.
4. Remove all visible fat from your occasional piece of red meat.
5. Dine on poultry twice a week.
6. Dine on seafood twice a week.
7. Dine on dinners comprised exclusively of vegetables twice a week.
8. Dine on pasta once a week.
9. Eat cooked dried pasta. (Fresh pasta contains more fat grams.)
10. Eat only one serving of bread per day. (Pita bread is number one in my book.)
11. Enjoy fruits early in the day.
12. Use mustard, ketchup, Worcestershire sauce, lite soy sauce, Tabasco®, cocktail sauce, chili sauce and horseradish in small amounts as flavor enhancers.
13. Use your favorite fresh or dried herbs to flavor foods.
14. Use degreased homemade or fat-free canned chicken or turkey broth when cooking rice and certain vegetables.
15. Use balsamic vinegar or prepared fat-free salad dressings when marinating or tossing salads.
16. Substitute skim milk for whole milk.
17. Use fat-free mayonnaise, sour cream, yogurt, butter substitutes and cheeses.
18. Drink plenty of water as your number one beverage. You may drink fruit juices early in the day. Coffee, tea and diet sodas are also permissible. You may also enjoy an occasional alcoholic beverage, but moderation is the golden rule.
19. Enjoy a multitude of fresh vegetables, lentils and grains.
20. Keep sugar products to a minimum, as it is my understanding that sugar turns into fat. (Reduce or eliminate sugar products in my recipes if you are on a low-sugar diet.)
21. Reduce or eliminate salt in my recipes if you are on a low-sodium diet.

22. Exercise. (Remember, no healthy lifestyle plan will work without it. I recommend forty minutes of power walking per day.)

Don't

1. Eat butter or margarine.
2. Eat foods or salad dressings prepared with oil.
3. Eat mayonnaise.
4. Eat cheese.
5. Eat nuts.
6. Eat egg yolks.
7. Eat olives.
8. Eat avocados.
9. Consume whole milk, half-and-half or cream.
10. Eat more than one cup of cooked pasta and one cup of sauce on pasta nights. (This rule also applies to rice.)
11. Eat bread on the days you are having a cereal or bread product for breakfast.
12. Eat bread on the days you are having pasta, grits or a barley dish for dinner.
13. Eat red meat, organ meat, or ham products except for pork tenderloin. (You may occasionally indulge your carnivorous cravings but only after you have lost some weight. I had a steak one month into my diet.)
14. Eat dessert. (You may treat yourself from time to time after you have graduated to a maintenance program. I adore Breyers® Pralines and Cream fat-free ice cream. SnackWell's® Devil's Food fat-free cookies are also pretty good!)

The Menu Planning Guide

"Life" and "hectic" are almost interchangeable in today's lexicon. Your mind and your body may be telling you to get a grip on your eating habits, but your time is spent closing deals, carpooling children or rushing to your next meeting. Taking time to plan proper meals may not fit into your schedule. That is why I designed the following section. I wanted to ease you into your new regimen by freeing you from the time-consuming guesswork of menu planning. The advantage of spelling out what to eat when also provides you with a disciplined support system without having to pay a weekly weight loss center.

Is it essential to follow my day-to-day recommendations? No. Remember, this is your diet; some personal adjustments have to be made. Case in point: I was amused by my friend Ann's exclamation as she scanned my breakfast suggestions. "Crumpets just don't satisfy me," she said. If crumpets don't appeal to you, have a cup of no- or low-fat cereal with skim milk. But do not have fried eggs and bacon. Use common sense and *The Paty Plan* principles to plan your own meals.

Your personalization of my meal plan extends beyond taste preference. Everyone's body is different. I have a stepdaughter who is blessed with her mother's metabolism. They both burn fat and calories with the blink of an eye. Heredity was not as kind to me. I have to eat less than they do to lose weight. You will need to know your own body and set some of your own rules. If you are not losing weight by eating eight ounces of chicken, reduce your intake to six. If pasta nights put on weight, eat more fish. If my Seafood Lasagna lands heavily on your thighs, broil a piece of pink salmon. These are judgments for you to make as you become knowledgeable about your body's requirements and limitations.

Speaking of limitations, I learned that I could not shed pounds and eat three squares a day—that turtle instead of the hare metabolism of mine. My solution to this dilemma was and is to eat two strategically-placed meals during the day. Nutritionists would recoil in horror if I revealed the timing of my meals. Dietitians advocate the importance of a substantial breakfast and a light dinner in the evening. My advice will not disappoint them. If your schedule permits, go ahead and have dinner midday. But do not be concerned if that game plan does not work for you. New evidence supports the theory that what you eat is as important as when you eat it.

You should find my menu guide easy to follow. I first give you seven breakfast and seven lunch meal suggestions. I also provide you with an acceptable snack list, but please do not linger long on that page. From there I spell out fifty-six dinner menus based on the weekly two-chicken, two-fish, two-vegetable and one-pasta Paty Plan entrée premise. Lastly, I put together two sample weeks that incorporate my breakfast, lunch and dinner ideas.

As you peruse the subsequent pages, remember, feel free to create your own menus once you have a concrete perception of your own needs coupled with a sound knowledge of the fat content in food.

My advice is to have fruit for breakfast six days a week.

Sprinkle some blueberries on your cold or hot cereal. Research studies reveal that blueberries contain multiple medical benefits. Antioxidants, positive cardiovascular agents and prevention of night blindness are some of the attributes of this tasty colorful fruit.

Breakfast Suggestions

One

1. One-half grapefruit

Two

1. Toasted crumpet with one tablespoon jam
   or
2. One cup no-fat cereal with one-half cup skim milk

Three

1. One-half cantaloupe
   or
2. One-quarter honeydew melon

Four

1. One sliced banana with berries

Five

1. Fat-free yogurt

Six

1. A mixture of your favorite fresh fruit

Seven

1. One cup cream of wheat
   or
2. An occasional cup of oatmeal

Eat only one-half of a pita pocket sandwich for lunch or dinner if the pounds are not melting away when you consume a whole sandwich.

Are you experiencing a mid-afternoon slump on consommé days? Enjoy a satisfying glass of tomato juice around 4:00 P.M.

Recipes marked with an asterisk can be found in the recipe section of this book.

Luncheon Suggestions

One

1. A can of chilled or heated consommé with seven fat-free saltines and carrot sticks (Try to have this lunch twice a week during the early stage of your diet. These days are not easy but you will appreciate the results.)

Two

1. Turkey, Chicken, Tuna or Seafood Salad on Lettuce Leaves or in Pita Pockets *

Three

1. Assorted fresh fruit
   or
2. Fresh Fruit Salad *

Four

1. One-half can tomato aspic with one-half cup fat-free cottage cheese on a bed of lettuce
   or
2. One-half can tomato aspic with fresh or canned asparagus on a bed of lettuce

Five

1. Tossed Marinated Vegetables *
   or
2. Plate of steamed or raw vegetables with one large fat-free rice cake (You may dip vegetables in a fat-free salad dressing.)

Six

1. Chef salad with lettuce, fat-free turkey or ham and cut vegetables tossed with a fat-free dressing

   or

2. A pita pocket sandwich with fat-free meat slices or fat-free cheese slices with sliced tomatoes and onions spread with mustard

Seven

1. One cup Tomato Zucchini Soup*, Gazpacho*, Minestrone Soup* or Black Bean Soup* (Eat only the Minestrone or Black Bean Soup for lunch when you are having vegetables for your evening meal.)

Snacks

Do not overindulge in snacks between meals. You will simply add unwanted calories. Crave a snack? Go for a walk instead. But if you still need a nibble to sustain yourself, here is a short list of no- to low-fat morsels:

- Raw vegetables (carrots, celery, radishes, etc.)
- Vegetable juice
- Fresh fruit early in the day
- Air-popped popcorn (Sprinkle with your favorite seasoning.)
- Fat-free pretzels (I like to dip them in a little mustard.)
- Fat-free rice cakes

My favorite treat is a frozen banana. Peel a banana, put it in a freezer bag, and place in the freezer for several hours. When frozen, pull back bag and eat the banana like a popsicle. You will think you are devouring a bowl of rich ice cream!

The Eight-Week Dinner Plan

First Week Dinner Suggestions

Sunday

1. Sliced Roast Turkey Breast* with one tablespoon Hot Cranberry-Pineapple Chutney* or Apple-Onion-Cranberry Chutney*
2. Baked sweet potato
3. Fresh green beans

Monday

1. Black Beans with Rice* (one cup each)
2. Mixed salad greens with balsamic vinegar or Quick and Easy Italian Dressing*

Tuesday

1. Grilled or Broiled Fish* with lemon
2. Steamed broccoli
3. Sliced Cucumbers and Onions*

Wednesday

1. Braised Cabbage, Onions and Carrots*

Thursday

1. Steamed Mussels with Angel Hair Pasta* or Pasta Marinara*
2. Mock Caesar Salad*

Friday

1. Aunt Barbara's Tomato and Vegetable Aspic* on a bed of lettuce with one-half cup fat-free cottage cheese

2. Fresh asparagus
3. Sliced hearts of palm

Saturday

1. Parmesan Summer Squash*
2. Broiled Tomatoes*
3. Boston lettuce salad with chopped green peppers and sliced red onion topped with balsamic vinegar *or* fat-free dressing

I am recommending four vegetable nights during the first seven days of *The Paty Plan.* You will enjoy the psychological benefits of a solid week of weight loss.

To retain the vibrant green color of asparagus: place trimmed asparagus into boiling water. Cook until desired doneness. Drain asparagus and rinse immediately under cold water.

Remember, the important pasta serving rule of thumb: eat only one cup of cooked pasta topped with one cup of sauce. Keep this rule in mind with rice dishes such as Fish and Corn Creole* and Oriental Chicken and Rice.*

A second rule of thumb: have only one pasta dinner entrée or one grits entrée or one barley entrée during a seven-day period. The grits and the barley dishes act as a substitute for your pasta dinner night of the week.

A festive addition to grilled or broiled fish:

- Sauté a couple of chopped green onions in olive oil cooking spray.
- Stir in one chopped tomato or one-half can Italian-style stewed tomatoes, two tablespoons white wine, one teaspoon minced garlic and a dash of chili powder.
- Bring green onion, tomato and wine mixture to a boil.
- Reduce heat and add scallops.
- Cook scallops for about two minutes.
- Season with salt and pepper and spoon over grilled or broiled fish.

Delicious with saffron rice and sautéed spinach!

Second Week

Sunday

1. Braised Chicken and Vegetables Vino*

Monday

1. Baked Acorn Squash*
2. Two of your favorite non-starch vegetables

Tuesday

1. Linguine with Mushroom Stroganoff* *or* Parmesan Corn Grits*
2. Mixed salad greens with sliced tomatoes topped with balsamic vinegar *or* fat-free dressing

Wednesday

1. Grilled or Broiled Fish* with lemon
2. Steamed or grilled zucchini
3. Red Pepper Cole Slaw*

Thursday

1. Vegetable Rice Pilaf*
2. Two of your favorite non-starch vegetables

Friday

1. Grilled Rosemary Chicken Breast on a Bed of Fresh Spinach*
2. Eggplant Italiano*

Saturday

1. Seafood Salad*
2. Pickles

Eat plenty of beta carotene-rich sweet potatoes, spinach and carrots. Be sure to also incorporate in your diet copious amounts of vitamin C-loaded broccoli.

Have you reached a plateau? Do not be discouraged. There are times when one hits a roadblock and the pounds are not melting away at a rapid pace. When this occurs eat:

- One-half grapefruit for breakfast
- Mixed salad greens and cut vegetables with fat-free dressing for lunch
- Two halves tuna *or* seafood pita bread sandwich for dinner

Third Week

Sunday

1. Minestrone Soup*

Monday

1. Turkey Taco Ensalada*

Tuesday

1. Mashed Sweet Potatoes*
2. Brussel sprouts
3. Beets

Wednesday

1. Oven "Fried" Fish* with lemon
2. Fresh asparagus
3. Tomato and Yellow Pepper Salsa*

Thursday

1. Baked Chicken Chutney*
2. Florentine Rice*
3. Salad with balsamic vinegar *or* fat-free dressing

Friday

1. Veggie Pita Pizza*
2. Tossed Artichoke Heart and Tomato Salad with Creamy Chive Vinaigrette*

Saturday

1. Fish and Corn Creole* *or* Seafood Lasagna*
2. Mixed salad greens with balsamic vinegar *or* fat-free dressing

News Flash! A recent study stated that a low-fat diet was not healthy. Why? Researchers claimed that people were eating low-fat "junk" food in place of the recommended daily servings of fruit, vegetables and grains. Not so with *The Paty Plan*. I do not encourage the consumption of fat-free chips, cookies, ice cream, etc. Look over my menu suggestions and recipes and you will see a healthy low-fat plan.

Fourth Week

Sunday

1. Vegetable Stew*

Monday

1. Grilled or Broiled Fish* with lemon
2. Oven Grilled Vegetable Medley*
3. Salad with balsamic vinegar *or* fat-free dressing

Tuesday

1. Cauliflower au Gratin*
2. Sweet and Sour Carrots*
3. Green beans

Wednesday

1. Turkey Stroganoff*
2. Mixed greens with balsamic vinegar *or* fat-free dressing

Thursday

1. Boiled shrimp with cocktail sauce
2. Artichoke, Tomato and Corn Salad*

Friday

1. Eggplant Parmigiana*
2. Romaine lettuce hearts with balsamic vinegar *or* fat-free dressing

Saturday

1. Maple-Dijon Barbecue Chicken* *or* Pork Tenderloin with Maple-Dijon Barbecue Sauce*
2. Rice

3. Boston lettuce leaves with Mandarin orange sections, sliced mushrooms and sliced red onions topped with fat-free poppy-seed dressing

Add a spoonful of mango chutney to a prepared fat-free poppyseed dressing for an extra special salad topping.

Another quick weight loss hint: substitute non-starch vegetables when you see potatoes or rice on my menu-planning guide.

Have you entered another frustrating slow-reducing phase? Do not despair. Adopt the following pound-busting menu for a day:

- One-half cantaloupe for breakfast
- One cup hot chicken broth and assorted cut raw or cooked vegetables for lunch
- Two halves turkey pita pockets for dinner

Fifth Week

Sunday

1. Grilled or Broiled Fish* with lemon
2. Steamed broccoli
3. Tomato and Corn Salsa*

Monday

1. Italian Vegetable Stew*
2. Romaine lettuce hearts with balsamic vinegar *or* fat-free dressing

Tuesday

1. Oven "Fried" Chicken*
2. Zippy Italian Lima Beans*

Wednesday

1. Shrimp and Corn Chowder* *or* Corn Chowder*
2. Tomato Bruschetta*

Thursday

1. Broccoli Cheese Squares* *or* Scalloped Potatoes*
2. Two of your favorite non-starch vegetables

Friday

1. Creamy Italian Baked Ziti* *or* "Hungry Chef in a Hurry" Pasta*
2. Mixed salad greens with balsamic vinegar *or* fat-free dressing

Saturday

1. Turkey or Chicken Salad Pita Pocket Sandwich*
2. Pickles

Sixth Week

Sunday

1. Grilled or Broiled Pink Salmon on a bed of Red Pepper Coulis*
2. German "Fried Potatoes"* *or* Cajun New Potatoes*
3. Steamed broccoli or zucchini

Monday

1. Aunt Barbara's Tomato and Vegetable Aspic* on a bed of lettuce with one-half cup fat-free cottage cheese
2. Fresh asparagus
3. Sliced hearts of palm

Tuesday

1. Turkey Burger*
2. Uncreamed Onions*
3. Salad with sliced peppers, steamed sugar snap peas and raw carrots topped with balsamic vinegar *or* fat-free dressing
   or
   Oriental Chicken and Vegetables with Rice*

Wednesday

1. Tuna Pasta Salad*

To dress up steamed broccoli or asparagus: sauté sliced mushrooms or chopped red peppers in olive oil cooking spray and spoon on top of your green vegetable.

25

Thursday

1. Grilled or Broiled Fish* with lemon
2. Rice and Spinach Stuffed Tomatoes*
3. Cucumbers and Onions*

Friday

1. Three of your favorite non-starch vegetables

Saturday

1. Turkey Enchilada Casserole*
2. Mixed salad greens with balsamic vinegar *or* fat-free dressing

---

Do not forget the importance of calcium in your diet. I have a glass of skim milk with my evening meal. Fat-free yogurt is another excellent source of calcium.

Seventh Week

Sunday

1. Garlic Mashed Potatoes* *or* baked potato
2. Green beans
3. Sweet and Sour Carrots*

Monday

1. Grilled or Broiled Fish* with lemon
2. Steamed zucchini
3. Broiled Tomatoes*

Tuesday

1. Mushroom Stuffed Pasta Shells* *or* Grits with Shrimp Sauce*
2. Mixed greens with balsamic vinegar *or* fat-free dressing

Wednesday

1. Three of your favorite non-starch vegetables

Thursday

1. Georgia-Mex Chicken* *or* Chicken Supreme*
2. Rice
3. Salad with balsamic vinegar *or* fat-free dressing

Friday

1. Summer Salmon with Shrimp*

Saturday

1. Grilled Rosemary Chicken Breast on a Bed of Fresh Spinach*
2. Boston lettuce leaves with sliced tomatoes, artichoke hearts and sliced onions topped with balsamic vinegar *or* fat-free dressing

Are the readings on the scales going up instead of down or not moving at all? Try to jump start weight loss by eating:

- One cup of no-fat cereal with skim milk topped with one-half cup of berries for breakfast
- Seafood salad on a bed of lettuce for lunch
- Steamed vegetables for dinner

New studies reveal that the potassium found in raw fruit and vegetables can lower blood pressure and prevent strokes. So eat your bananas and uncooked veggies! Tomatoes and spinach also top the anti-stroke chart.

Eighth Week

Sunday

1. Tuna Pita Sandwich*
2. Pickles

Monday

1. Chicken and Wild Rice Salad* *or* Corn, Rice and Black Bean Salad*

Tuesday

1. Parmesan Summer Squash*
2. Green beans
3. Salad with raw vegetables topped with balsamic vinegar *or* fat-free dressing

Wednesday

1. Turkey, Barley, Vegetable Soup* *or* Mushroom Barley Risotto*
2. Mixed salad greens with balsamic vinegar *or* fat-free dressing

Thursday

1. Poached Fish Rossa with New Potatoes*
2. Romaine lettuce hearts with sliced red onions topped with balsamic vinegar *or* fat-free dressing

Friday

1. Three of your favorite non-starch vegetables

Saturday

1. Great Northern Bean and Spinach Gratin* *or* Seafood Florentine*

The Two-Week Menu Guide

First Week Breakfast, Lunch and Dinner Menu Suggestions

Sunday

A. Breakfast
   1. One-half cantaloupe

B. Lunch
   1. One can chilled or heated consommé
   2. Seven fat-free saltines
   3. Carrot sticks

C. Dinner
   1. Sliced Roast Turkey Breast* with one tablespoon Hot Cranberry Pineapple Chutney* *or* Apple-Onion-Cranberry Chutney*
   2. Baked sweet potato
   3. Fresh green beans

Monday

A. Breakfast
   1. Assorted fresh fruit

B. Lunch
   1. Tossed Marinated Vegetables*

C. Dinner
   1. Black Beans with Rice*
   2. Mixed salad greens with balsamic vinegar *or* Quick and Easy Italian Dressing*

Tuesday

A. Breakfast
   1. Sliced bananas and berries

B. Lunch
   1. One cup Tomato-Zucchini Soup*

C. Dinner
   1. Grilled or Broiled Fish* with lemon
   2. Steamed broccoli
   3. Sliced Cucumbers and Onions*

Wednesday

A. Breakfast
   1. One-quarter honeydew melon

B. Lunch
   1. One-half pita sandwich of choice

C. Dinner
   1. Braised Cabbage, Carrots and Onions*

Thursday

A. Breakfast
   1. One-half grapefruit

B. Lunch
   1. One can chilled or heated consommé
   2. Seven fat-free saltines
   3. Carrot sticks

C. Dinner
   1. Steamed Mussels with Angel Hair Pasta* *or* Pasta Marinara*
   2. Mock Caesar Salad*

Friday

A. Breakfast
   1. One cup no-fat cereal with one-half cup skim milk

B. Lunch
   1. Tuna or Seafood Salad* on lettuce

C. Dinner
   1. Aunt Barbara's Tomato and Vegetable Aspic* on a bed of lettuce with one-half cup fat-free cottage cheese
   2. Fresh asparagus
   3. Sliced hearts of palm

Saturday

A. Breakfast
   1. Melon and berries

B. Lunch
   1. Plate of steamed or raw vegetables
   2. One large fat-free rice cake

C. Dinner
   1. Parmesan Summer Squash*
   2. Broiled Tomatoes*
   3. Boston lettuce salad with chopped green peppers and sliced red onion topped with balsamic vinegar *or* fat-free dressing

Second Week Breakfast, Lunch and Dinner Menu Suggestions

Sunday

A. Breakfast
   1. One-half cantaloupe

B. Lunch
   1. Tossed Marinated Vegetables*

C. Dinner
   1. Braised Chicken and Vegetables Vino*

Monday

A. Breakfast
   1. Crumpet with one tablespoon jam

B. Lunch
   1. Chef salad with lettuce, fat-free turkey and cut vegetables tossed with a fat-free dressing

C. Dinner
   1. Baked Acorn Squash*
   2. Two of your favorite non-starch vegetables

Tuesday

A. Breakfast
   1. Assorted Fruit

B. Lunch
   1. One can chilled or heated consommé
   2. Seven fat-free saltines
   3. Carrot sticks

C. Dinner
1. Linguine with Mushroom Stroganoff* *or* Parmesan Corn Grits*
2. Mixed salad greens with sliced tomatoes topped with balsamic vinegar *or* fat-free dressing

Wednesday

A. Breakfast
1. One-quarter honeydew melon

B. Lunch
1. One-half canned tomato aspic on a bed of lettuce with one-half cup fat-free cottage cheese *or* with asparagus

C. Dinner
1. Grilled or Broiled Fish* with lemon
2. Steamed or grilled zucchini
3. Red Pepper Cole Slaw*

Thursday

A. Breakfast
1. Fat-free yogurt

B. Lunch
1. Fresh Fruit Salad*

C. Dinner
1. Vegetable Rice Pilaf*
2. Two of your favorite non-starch vegetables

Friday

A. Breakfast
1. One-half grapefruit

B. Lunch
1. Gazpacho*

C. Dinner
1. Grilled Rosemary Chicken Breast on a Bed of Fresh Spinach*
2. Eggplant Italiano*

Saturday

A. Breakfast
1. Banana and berries

B. Lunch
1. Plate of steamed or raw vegetables
2. One large fat-free rice cake

C. Dinner
1. Seafood Salad*
2. Pickles

The Recipes

While many of my busy fast- and fat-food addicted friends were excited to learn that I was writing this book, all expressed a common concern: "Please make the recipes simple," they pleaded. I heeded their words. The recipes in the next chapter are dedicated to all the people living in our frenetic workaday world. My non-cooking friends will be equally happy to learn that one does not have to be overly kitchen literate to whip up my low-fat concoctions. Time constraints and ignorance can no longer be excuses for poor eating habits.

We live in an age when adhering to my "diet" and creating low-fat meals is no longer a challenge. While new products on the market have helped create this environment, I do realize you may find it difficult to acclimate yourself to the much-maligned fat-free cheeses, sour cream, mayonnaise and butters. While it is vital to abstain from the Real McCoy, you may choose to delete the fat-free imitations from my recipes. Let your own taste buds be your advisor on this matter.

As you head to the kitchen to prepare my recipes, it is essential to keep that last notion in mind. Your personal culinary preferences are important. While my favorite meals are heavily infused with chili powder and cumin, you might prefer curry powder and saffron. It is also no secret that I adore Italian cuisine, but foods with an Oriental influence might be your favorite choice. Feel free to put your personal signature on my recipes as long as you remain steadfast to the principles of *The Paty Plan*. Your imagination should be your guide as you incorporate my weight loss formula into your lifetime commitment to healthy eating habits.

Tuna Pita Bread Sandwich

Serves one to two

1 6 ⅛-ounce can tuna in water,
  drained
1 teaspoon chopped red onion
  or to taste
1 stick celery, coarsely
  chopped

1 small tomato, chopped
1 teaspoon sweet relish
1 tablespoon Dijon mustard
1 6-inch individual loaf pita
  bread, cut in half

- Combine first five ingredients with Dijon mustard.
- Spoon tuna mixture into pita bread pockets.

Turkey or Chicken Salad Pita Pocket Sandwich

Serves one to two

¾ cup cooked turkey or chicken breast, diced
1 celery stick, chopped
2 green onions, chopped or chopped red onion to taste
1 cup leaf lettuce, shredded
2 fresh basil leaves, chopped or fresh tarragon to taste

2 teaspoons fat-free sour cream
2 teaspoons Dijon mustard
½ teaspoon red wine vinegar
dash of salt and freshly ground pepper
1 6-inch individual loaf pita bread, cut in half

- Combine together first five ingredients.
- Whisk together sour cream, mustard and vinegar.
- Toss sour cream mixture with salad.
- Season salad with salt and pepper.
- Spoon salad mixture into pita bread pockets.

Seafood Salad

Serves one to two

1 8-ounce package Louis
  Kemp® Crab or Lobster
  Delights
2 spring onions, chopped
1 stalk celery, chopped
1 small tomato, diced
1 to 2 tablespoons fresh basil,
  chopped

¾ teaspoon fresh chive,
  chopped
salt and pepper
1 tablespoon fat-free sour
  cream
1 teaspoon Dijon mustard
1 teaspoon red wine vinegar
½ teaspoon fresh lemon juice
pita bread or lettuce leaves

- Combine first six ingredients and season with salt and pepper.
- Whisk together sour cream, mustard, vinegar and lemon juice.
- Toss sour cream mixture with crab mixture and adjust seasonings.
- Serve in pita pockets or on a bed of lettuce.

Fresh Fruit Salad

Serves one

¼ sliced mango
¼ cup pineapple chunks
½ cup grape halves

Lime wedge
Boston lettuce

- In a bowl, toss together the fresh fruit and squeeze with the lime.
- Serve on a bed of lettuce.

Is tonight a vegetable night? If it is, add two ounces of cubed turkey breast to above for lunch. This salad does not require dressing due to the lusciousness of the fruit.

For a nice fruit salad alternative: toss together fresh spinach or Boston lettuce, Mandarin orange sections, sliced mushrooms and red onion with a little raspberry vinegar and lime juice or a prepared fat-free poppyseed dressing. Add two crumbled pieces of cooked turkey bacon for a delicious poultry dinner salad.

Tossed Marinated Vegetables

Serves four

1 14-ounce can artichoke hearts, drained and quartered

1 14-ounce can hearts of palm, drained and sliced

1 pint cherry tomatoes, halved or quartered

2 green onions, sliced

4 tablespoons prepared fat-free salad dressing

salt and pepper

- Mix together all ingredients.
- Cover and chill for one hour.
- Serve in salad bowl or on a bed of lettuce.

Tomato Zucchini Soup

Serves two

2 cups fat-free chicken broth	1 14½-ounce can Italian style
2 large zucchini, sliced	stewed tomatoes
1 onion, sliced	1 teaspoon minced garlic
	salt, pepper and chili powder
	to taste

- Place all ingredients in a saucepan.
- Bring ingredients to a boil.
- Reduce to a medium heat and cook until all vegetables are tender.
- Place soup in a blender and purée until smooth.
- Return puréed mixture to the saucepan, adjust seasonings and reheat.
- Serve with fat-free Parmesan cheese.

Another simple soup idea:

- Sauté eight ounces of sliced mushrooms in olive oil cooking spray.
- Sauté three chopped green onions in cooking spray.
- Spoon one can low-fat cream of mushroom soup into a saucepan.
- Stir in mushrooms, green onions, one cup skim milk, three tablespoons no-fat sour cream, two tablespoons Madeira wine, one teaspoon Dijon mustard, salt, pepper and a dash of chili powder.
- Cook soup mixture over medium heat until all ingredients are well-combined and hot. *Serves three*.

Delete all but a little skim milk and this creamy mushroom mixture makes a delicious sauce spooned over grilled chicken breasts.

Minestrone Soup

Serves two

2 cups fat-free chicken broth
2 carrots, peeled and diced
1 14½-ounce can Italian style
    stewed tomatoes
½ cup red kidney beans

1 zucchini, diced
¾ cup dry rotelle pasta
salt, pepper, garlic powder,
    chili powder and dried
    oregano to taste

- Place the first two ingredients in a saucepan.
- Bring the broth and carrots to a boil.
- Reduce to a medium heat and cook carrots until crisp tender.
- Add the tomatoes, kidney beans, zucchini and seasonings.
- Return to high heat and cook until the zucchini is almost tender.
- Add the rotelle and boil until pasta is done. Avoid overcooking the pasta.
- Adjust seasonings and serve with fat-free Parmesan cheese.

Black Bean Soup

Serves two

1 15-ounce can black beans,
    undrained
1 14½-ounce can Italian style
    stewed tomatoes
1 to 2 cups fat-free chicken
    broth
1 onion, chopped

1 teaspoon minced garlic
salt, pepper, chili powder to
    taste
cumin to taste
chopped green onions and
    fat-free sour cream (op-
    tional)

- Mix together in a saucepan the beans, tomatoes, one cup broth, onions and seasonings.
- Bring the mixture to a boil.
- Reduce heat and simmer one hour.
- While simmering, add more chicken broth if the soup becomes too thick.
- Place the simmered mixture in a blender and purée for a few seconds.
- Return the puréed soup to the saucepan, adjust seasonings and reheat.
- Serve with chopped green onions and fat-free sour cream.

Add about one tablespoon instant mashed potatoes to thicken any soup or sauce.

Gazpacho

Serves two

1 cup tomato juice or V8® vegetable
juice
1 cup prepared chunky salsa
1 tomato, chopped
1 cucumber, peeled and
chopped

½ yellow bell pepper,
chopped
2 green onions, sliced
1 teaspoon Dijon mustard
1 tablespoon balsamic vinegar
salt and pepper

- Combine all the ingredients in a bowl.
- Cover the bowl and refrigerate for at least one hour.
- Serve topped with a dash of Tabasco® and a dollop of fat-free sour cream.

Want a special treat?
Mix in six ounces of baby shrimp.

Roasted Turkey Breast and Stock

1 6-pound turkey breast   salt and cracked black pepper
                                           3 cups water

- Preheat oven to 325 degrees.
- Place seasoned turkey breast in a large roasting pan.
- Place three cups of water in bottom of the roasting pan.
- Roast turkey for about 2½ hours or until meat thermometer registers 180 degrees. Baste every 30 minutes.
- Remove turkey from oven and let rest for 15 minutes before slicing.

For stock:

- Place cooled turkey stock liquid into a plastic container.
- Chill cooled stock in refrigerator until the fat congeals on the surface.
- Spoon fat off stock.
- Refrigerate for two to three days or freeze.

A couple of helpful hints: add more water to pan while roasting if water evaporates. Use this tasty stock instead of water to boil potatoes or to cook rice or vegetables.

To prepare chicken stock: place an uncooked and cut-up chicken in a large pot. Cover the chicken with water and add one chopped onion, two chopped celery stalks, two bay leaves and several peppercorns. Bring to a boil, lower heat and simmer for three hours. Be sure to skim the scum off the top as chicken simmers. Strain the stock and cool. Save the skinned chicken parts for dinner or another recipe. Place the stock in the refrigerator and chill until the fat congeals. Spoon the fat off the surface and return to the refrigerator until utilized. Use within three days or freeze up to six months.

Hot Cranberry-Pineapple Chutney

Serves eight

1 16-ounce can whole-berry
   cranberry sauce, drained

1 8¼-ounce can crushed pineapple, drained
2 to 5 ounces prepared horseradish

• Mix together all ingredients and chill.

Apple-Onion-Cranberry Chutney

Serves six

Cooking spray
2 yellow onions, thinly sliced
3 Granny Smith apples,
   peeled, cored and cut into
   chunks

4 tablespoons apple cider
   vinegar
3 tablespoons brown sugar
1 teaspoon cinnamon
1 16-ounce can whole-berry
   cranberry sauce

- In a nonstick saucepan, sprayed with cooking spray, sauté the onions until soft.
- Stir in the next four ingredients and one-half of the cranberry sauce.
- Bring the mixture to a boil, reduce heat and simmer for 25 minutes.
- Drain the chutney and return it to the saucepan.
- Stir in the remaining cranberry sauce and continue to simmer for 10 minutes.
- Serve warm or at room temperature.

You will think you are in heaven if you place the Apple-Onion-Cranberry Chutney over a grilled chicken breast.

Black Beans and Rice

Serves three to four

olive oil cooking spray
1 cup onion, chopped
1 red pepper, chopped
2 15-ounce cans black beans,
 drained
1 14½-ounce can Italian style
 stewed tomatoes
1 cup fat-free chicken broth
1 8-ounce can tomato sauce

2 tablespoons tomato paste
2 teaspoons minced garlic
chili powder to taste
cumin to taste
salt and pepper
4 cups cooked rice
chopped green onions (op-
 tional)

- Spray a large nonstick skillet with cooking spray.
- Add the onions and red peppers and sauté until soft.
- Stir in the next eight ingredients and season with salt and pepper.
- Bring the mixture to a boil, reduce heat and simmer for one hour.
- Adjust seasonings and serve over one cup of hot rice. Top with green onions, if desired.

Prepare recipes with garlic, garlic and more garlic. Healers from history and current day researchers claim that the consumption of this bulb plant has positive health benefits.

Quick and Easy Italian Dressing

2 tablespoons balsamic vinegar

2 tablespoons red wine vinegar with garlic

1 1.05-ounce package Good Seasons® fat-free Italian dressing

3 tablespoons water

½ teaspoon minced garlic

½ teaspoon prepared horseradish

1 teaspoon Dijon mustard

¼ teaspoon anchovy paste

½ cup water

- Place first four ingredients in a jar with a tight lid and shake vigorously.
- Add remaining ingredients and shake again until well-blended.
- Dressing may be refrigerated for up to one month.

Grilled or Broiled Fish

Serves two

1 pound pink salmon fillet,
    grouper fillet, swordfish
    or your favorite white
    fish
salt and pepper

½ lemon
fresh dill, chive or your
    favorite herbs
extra lemon wedges

- Prepare grill to medium-high heat or preheat broiler.
- Squeeze lemon evenly over fish and sprinkle both sides with your favorite chopped herbs.
- Season both sides of fish with salt and pepper.
- Grill or broil fish for about five minutes per side or until just opaque in the center.

A special treat is to place your fish on a bed of the following red pepper coulis: sauté two finely chopped red bell peppers and two finely chopped shallots until soft in a nonstick saucepan sprayed with olive oil cooking spray. Stir in and bring to a boil one cup fat-free chicken broth, one teaspoon minced garlic and one tablespoon canned chopped green chilies. Partially cover, reduce heat and simmer for 25 minutes. Place red pepper mixture in a processor and blend until smooth. Return puréed sauce to saucepan, add one tablespoon balsamic vinegar, salt and pepper and spoon warm coulis on a plate and top with grilled or broiled fish.

My favorite side dish with grilled fish is sliced cucumbers combined with sliced red onion and tossed with balsamic vinegar.

Braised Cabbage, Onions and Carrots

Serves two

4 carrots, peeled and sliced
    lengthwise
2 onions, quartered
1 14½-ounce can Italian style
    stewed tomatoes
¼ cup red wine
2 tablespoons balsamic vine-
    gar

garlic powder, chili powder,
    and cumin
½ cabbage, cored and cut into
    large wedges
2 cups fat-free chicken broth
1 cup water
salt and pepper

- Preheat oven to 325 degrees.
- Place carrots and onions in a baking dish.
- Pour the tomatoes, wine and vinegar over vegetables and season with garlic, chili powder, cumin, salt and pepper.
- Cover baking dish with foil and bake vegetables for a couple of hours or until tender.
- While carrots and onions are braising, bring the chicken broth and water to a boil and add the cabbage.
- Season cabbage with salt and pepper and cook for about 15 minutes or until crisp-tender and drain.
- Serve hot vegetables with juices from the baking dish.

In a rush? Parboil the carrots and onions and reduce baking time in half.

To make a delicious marinara sauce: spray a deep skillet or saucepan with olive oil cooking spray and sauté one chopped onion until soft. Stir in two 14½-ounce cans Italian-style stewed tomatoes, one cup red wine, ¾ cup fat-free chicken broth, one 6-ounce can tomato paste, two teaspoons minced garlic, one teaspoon dried oregano, ½ package Equal®, chili powder, salt and pepper to taste. Bring the mixture to a boil. Reduce heat and simmer for 45 minutes. Add two tablespoons of chopped fresh basil and serve over your favorite cooked pasta. *Serves four.*

You do not need oil to prevent pasta from sticking together. Instead, swirl boiling pasta with tongs several times while cooking.

Steamed Mussels with Angel Hair Pasta

Serves four

olive oil cooking spray
2 shallots, chopped
1 teaspoon minced garlic
1 cup dry vermouth
2 pounds live pre-soaked and
   debearded mussels

2 14½-ounce cans Italian style
   stewed tomatoes
⅓ cup fresh basil, chopped
salt to taste, pepper to taste,
   chili powder to taste
½ pound dried angel hair
   pasta

- Sauté shallots in 4-quart stockpot sprayed with cooking spray. Do not burn.
- Add garlic, vermouth and mussels.
- Cover pan and steam mussels over high heat for five minutes or until mussels are open. Shake pan several times while mussels are cooking.
- Remove mussels with tongs to a heated bowl.
- Add tomatoes, basil and seasonings to wine stock.
- Bring to a hard boil. Reduce heat and simmer ten minutes or until sauce thickens.
- Cook angel hair pasta according to package directions and drain while sauce is simmering.
- Put pasta into individual bowls. Place mussels around pasta and spoon sauce over angel hair pasta and mussels.
- Serve with fat-free Parmesan cheese.

Mock Caesar Salad

Serves four

⅓ cup red wine vinegar
¾ teaspoon anchovy paste
1 teaspoon minced garlic
2 teaspoons Dijon mustard
¼ teaspoon Worcestershire
    sauce
¼ teaspoon prepared horse-
    radish

1 tablespoon fat-free grated
    Parmesan cheese
dash Tabasco®
salt and freshly cracked pep-
    per to taste
1 head romaine lettuce, torn
1 cup fat-free garlic croutons

- Whisk together first nine ingredients.
- Place lettuce and croutons in a large salad bowl, toss with dressing and serve immediately.

To make creamy Caesar Salad dressing: add one tablespoon fat-free sour cream to first nine ingredients.

Your lips will surely pucker with this Caesar Salad dressing. Add a pinch or two of sugar or a dash of Equal® if you want to cut the tartness.

Aunt Barbara's Tomato and Vegetable Aspic

Serves four as a main dish
Serves six to eight as a side dish

1½ envelopes unflavored gela-
    tin
1½ tablespoons white vinegar
1 Equal® packet
2 14½-ounce cans stewed to-
    matoes, regular or Italian
    style

½ cup yellow or green pepper,
    chopped
½ cup celery, chopped
½ cup onion, chopped
½ teaspoon salt
½ to 1 tablespoon prepared
    horseradish (optional)
olive oil cooking spray

- Mix together first three ingredients.
- Heat tomatoes in a saucepan.
- Stir together the gelatin mixture and tomatoes.
- Add remaining ingredients and mix well.
- Pour into a 2-quart mold sprayed with cooking spray and chill until firm.
- Serve on a bed of lettuce with fat-free cottage cheese, if desired.

Parmesan Summer Squash

Serves two to four

1½ cups water
1½ pounds summer squash,
    trimmed and sliced
1 onion, peeled and sliced

¼ cup grated fat-free Parmesan cheese
salt and pepper to taste

- Bring the water to a boil, add the squash and onions and cook over a medium heat until tender.
- Drain the squash and return it to the saucepan.
- Add the Parmesan cheese and seasonings.
- Mix the ingredients together over a low heat until hot.

Broiled Tomatoes

Serves four

olive oil cooking spray
2 large tomatoes, each cut into
    four thick slices
¼ cup Italian style bread
    crumbs

2 tablespoons fat-free Parme-
    san cheese
garlic powder, dried oregano,
    salt and pepper to taste

- Place tomatoes on a sheet pan sprayed with olive oil cooking spray.
- Evenly top each tomato slice with the bread crumbs and fat-free Parmesan cheese.
- Sprinkle each tomato slice with garlic powder, dried oregano, salt and pepper.
- Broil until lightly browned or bake in a 350 degree oven for 15 minutes.

Braised Chicken and Vegetables Vino

Serves two

2 chicken leg quarters, all skin and fat removed
6 carrots, peeled and cut lengthwise
2 unpeeled potatoes, quartered or 4 new potatoes
2 onions, peeled and halved with root intact

1 14½-ounce can Italian style stewed tomatoes
¼ cup balsamic vinegar
¼ cup red wine
salt, pepper, garlic powder, ground cumin and chili powder *or* salt, pepper, garlic powder, dried rosemary and dried oregano

- Preheat oven to 325 degrees.
- Place chicken in the middle of a roasting pan.
- Place vegetables around the chicken.
- Pour tomatoes, vinegar and wine over chicken and vegetables.
- Generously season all ingredients.
- Cover pan tightly with aluminum foil.
- Braise in oven for 2 hours or until chicken and vegetables are tender.
- Serve with pan juices.

I bake this dish for two hours, as I like my chicken meat to fall off the bone. It sometimes takes the vegetables even longer to cook. If so, remove the cooked chicken and continue to bake the vegetables until tender or parboil the vegetables for about seven minutes before baking.

Baked Acorn Squash

Serves two

1 acorn squash, halved and
   seeded

2 teaspoons brown sugar
salt and pepper to taste

- Preheat oven to 400 degrees.
- Pour enough water into baking dish to fill it about one inch deep.
- Set squash halves cut side down in dish.
- Cover the dish with aluminum foil and bake 45 minutes or until squash is tender.
- Remove dish from oven and turn squash so cut sides face upward.
- Sprinkle squash halves with brown sugar, salt and pepper.
- Return squash to oven and bake uncovered an additional 10 to 15 minutes.

Serve your guests the cooked acorn squash filled with peas. The contrasting orange and green hues make for a colorful presentation with a nice marriage of flavors.

In the mood for pasta and seafood? Sauté a couple of chopped green onions in olive oil cooking spray. Add a few tablespoons of white wine. Bring wine and green onions to a boil. Reduce heat and add some scallops. Cook scallops for about two minutes. Season with salt and pepper. Toss the scallops into the mushroom sauce and spoon mixture over cooked linguine.

Do not forget pasta and rice lovers: eat one cup of pasta or rice to one cup of sauce.

Linguine with Mushrooms Stroganoff

Serves four

olive oil cooking spray
2 pounds mushrooms, sliced
1 teaspoon minced garlic or to
    taste
1 cup cold skim milk
2 tablespoons Wondra® quick
    mixing flour
½ cup white wine or Madeira
    wine
¼ cup fat-free sour cream

2 teaspoons Dijon mustard or
    to taste
1 teaspoon tomato paste
salt, freshly cracked pepper
    and chili powder to taste
2 tablespoons fresh chive,
    chopped
12 ounces linguine, cooked
    and drained

- Sauté mushrooms until tender in a deep nonstick skillet sprayed with cooking spray.
- Stir in garlic.
- Mix together milk and flour and add to mushrooms.
- Add wine and cook over a medium heat for about four minutes.
- Stir in sour cream, mustard, tomato paste and seasonings and cook over a low heat for an additional five minutes.
- Spoon sauce over linguine and top with chive.
- Serve with fat-free grated Parmesan cheese.

Parmesan Corn Grits

Serves three to four

2 cups water
2 cups fat-free chicken broth
1 cup quick grits
2 ears of corn, cooked and cut
off the cob
1 8½-ounce can cream style
corn

¼ cup skim milk
4 tablespoons fat-free Parmesan cheese
salt and pepper to taste
paprika
cut fresh chive (optional)

- Put the water and chicken broth in a saucepan.
- Bring the liquid to a boil and slowly stir in the grits.
- Reduce heat to low and cover the saucepan.
- Cook the grits for about seven minutes or until thickened. Be sure to stir occasionally while cooking.
- Stir in the next four ingredients and generously season with salt and pepper.
- Serve hot grits topped with paprika and fresh chive, if desired.

Red Pepper Cole Slaw

Serves four

5 cups cabbage, coarsely
    chopped
½ red bell pepper, chopped
3 tablespoons red onion,
    chopped
1 heaping tablespoon sweet
    relish
¼ cup fat-free sour cream

1 tablespoon Dijon mustard
1 tablespoon red wine vinegar
¼ teaspoon minced garlic
¼ teaspoon anchovy paste
1 teaspoon prepared horse-
    radish
salt and freshly ground pep-
    per to taste

- In a bowl, combine first four ingredients.
- In a separate bowl, make dressing by whisking together the next six ingredients.
- Toss dressing with cabbage mixture and add seasonings.
- Serve immediately or chill one hour.

Vegetable Rice Pilaf

Serves six

olive oil cooking spray
1 medium onion, finely
    chopped
2 stalks celery, finely chopped
1 cup uncooked rice
1 cup frozen peas, thawed
12 ounces fresh mushrooms,
    sliced and sautéed

or

1 8-ounce can sliced mush-
    rooms
1 14½-ounce can fat-free
    chicken broth
¼ cup water or white wine
salt and pepper to taste

- Preheat oven to 350 degrees.
- Sauté onion and celery until soft in a nonstick skillet.
- Add rice and sauté with onions and celery for two minutes.
- Stir peas and mushrooms into rice mixture.
- Meanwhile heat together broth and water or wine to boiling.
- Stir boiling liquid into rice mixture and add salt and pepper.
- Transfer rice and vegetables to a 1½-quart casserole.
- Bake covered for 45 minutes or until all liquid is absorbed.

Add a small amount of water to your pan if vegetables are sticking when sautéing with olive oil cooking spray.

Grilled Rosemary Chicken Breasts on a Bed of Fresh Spinach

Serves four

2 large chicken breasts, skinned and boned
salt and freshly ground pepper
¼ teaspoon poultry seasoning
¼ cup distilled white vinegar
1 tablespoon honey
1 teaspoon lemon juice
1 tablespoon fresh rosemary
2 tablespoons fresh chive, chopped
2 green onions, chopped and sautéed in olive oil cooking spray
12 ounces fresh spinach, washed and dried
2 teaspoons minced garlic
additional salt and pepper
olive oil cooking spray

- Place chicken in a nonmetallic shallow dish.
- Season both sides of chicken with salt, pepper and poultry seasoning.
- In a small bowl, whisk together vinegar, lemon juice and honey.
- Pour vinegar marinade over chicken and top each piece with rosemary, chive and onions.
- Marinate chicken in refrigerator for three hours, basting every hour.
- Remove chicken from refrigerator and let it sit at room temperature for an additional hour.
- Prepare grill for medium heat.
- Grill chicken seven to ten minutes per side.
- While chicken is still grilling, spray a large nonstick skillet with olive oil spray.
- Place spinach in the skillet and add garlic, salt and pepper.
- Tossing constantly, cook spinach over a medium heat until wilted.*
- Divide spinach evenly on four plates.
- Top spinach with one-half cooked chicken breast.

*May need to be done in two batches.

Eggplant Italiano

Serves four

olive oil cooking spray
1 eggplant, peeled and cut
    into eight ½-inch slices
⅓ cup Italian style bread
    crumbs
16 fresh basil leaves

2 tomatoes, sliced
salt, pepper and garlic pow-
    der to taste
8 slices fat-free mozzarella
    cheese

- Preheat broiler.
- Spray nonstick baking sheet with cooking spray.
- Put bread crumbs in a shallow bowl.
- Lightly spray each cut side of eggplant with cooking spray and coat each side in bread crumbs.
- Place eggplant on baking sheet and broil for four minutes per side or until brown.
- Place two basil leaves on each eggplant slice after it has cooled.
- Top basil with tomato slice.
- Season top of tomato with salt, pepper and garlic powder and cover with mozzarella.
- Broil until cheese melts.

Turkey Taco Ensalada

Serves four

olive oil cooking spray
1½ pounds ground turkey
  breast
salt, pepper, garlic powder,
  ground cumin and chili
  powder to taste
2 19-ounce cans black beans,
  partially drained
1 15.25-ounce can whole ker-
  nel corn, drained
1 8-ounce can tomato sauce
1½ cups chunky salsa, divided
  into one cup and one-half
  cup

6 cups romaine lettuce hearts,
  torn
2 tomatoes, coarsely chopped
½ cup red onion, sliced
⅓ cup fat-free creamy ranch
  dressing
1 cup grated fat-free cheddar
  cheese
6 scallions, thinly sliced
4 servings low-fat baked
  Tostitos® (13 per plate)

- Sauté ground turkey breast in a large nonstick skillet sprayed generously with olive oil cooking spray.
- Season ground turkey with salt, pepper, garlic powder, ground cumin and chili powder.
- Add beans, corn, tomato sauce, one cup salsa and mix together.
- Add more seasonings to taste.
- Simmer uncovered for 45 minutes.
- While turkey mixture is simmering, combine lettuce, tomatoes and onion in a large bowl.
- Combine in a small bowl one-half cup salsa and ranch dressing.
- Pour dressing over lettuce mixture and toss.
- Spoon turkey mixture over lettuce.
- Sprinkle cheese and scallions over lettuce and turkey mixture.
- Place chips around salad and serve immediately.

Mashed Sweet Potatoes

Serves four to six

4 sweet potatoes, scrubbed
    and halved or quartered
½ cup orange juice
¼ cup skim milk

2 teaspoons brown sugar
¼ teaspoon cinnamon
salt to taste
butter-flavored cooking spray

- Place potatoes in a pot of water and bring to a boil.
- Reduce heat and cook potatoes for 30 to 60 minutes or until tender.
- Drain potatoes, cool slightly and peel.
- Mash the potatoes with a manual masher or electric mixer.
- Stir in orange juice, skim milk, brown sugar, cinnamon and salt and mix well.
- Put the mashed potatoes in a baking dish sprayed with cooking spray and bake in a preheated 350 degree oven for 30 minutes or until hot and bubbly.

Oven "Fried" Chicken

Serves four

4 chicken breast halves,
   skinned and boned
2 tablespoons Dijon mustard
2 tablespoons fat-free sour
   cream
¾ cup Italian style bread
   crumbs

2 tablespoons fat-free grated
   Parmesan cheese
⅛ teaspoon garlic powder
⅛ teaspoon chili powder
¼ teaspoon dried oregano
1 tablespoon dried parsley
salt and pepper to taste
olive oil cooking spray

- Preheat oven to 375 degrees.
- Whisk together mustard and sour cream.
- Combine bread crumbs, cheese, garlic powder, chili powder, oregano and parsley in a bowl and mix together.
- Season chicken liberally with salt and pepper.
- Spread Dijon mixture evenly over chicken sides.
- Coat all sides of chicken pieces in bread crumb mixture.
- Place chicken on a baking sheet sprayed with cooking spray.
- Spray top of chicken lightly with cooking spray and bake for 30 to 35 minutes.

For Oven "Fried" Fish: substitute boneless white fish for chicken and bake for about 20 minutes. For an extra crispy version: turn oven up to 400 degrees during the last five minutes of baking.

Tomato and Yellow Pepper Salsa

Serves four

3 medium tomatoes, chopped
  coarsely
1 yellow pepper, chopped
½ small red onion, chopped
  finely
2 tablespoons chopped green
  chilies

2 tablespoons fresh basil,
  chopped
2 tablespoons Italian parsley
  or cilantro, chopped
dash of salt, pepper and
  cumin
2 tablespoons balsamic vinegar

- Stir together all ingredients in a bowl and serve.

If preparing this recipe in advance, do not add balsamic
vinegar until serving time.

Baked Chicken Chutney

Serves two

2 chicken breast halves,
    skinned and boned

2 heaping tablespoons mango
    chutney
salt and pepper to taste
water

- Preheat oven to 350 degrees.
- Season both sides of chicken with salt and pepper.
- Place chicken breasts in a baking pan.
- Spread the mango chutney evenly over the top of the chicken breasts.
- Place a little water in the bottom of the pan.
- Bake chicken for 30 minutes or until done.
- Serve pan juices over rice, if desired.

> It is no secret that boning and skinning chicken breasts is not my favorite pastime. I spend a little more money and buy my chicken breasts ready for the pan. I know that Martha and Natalie would not be proud of me!

Florentine Rice

Serves six

2½ cups canned fat-free chicken broth or home-made chicken or turkey stock
1 cup uncooked rice

1 10-ounce package frozen chopped spinach, cooked and drained*
salt and pepper to taste

- Bring chicken broth to a boil in a medium saucepan.
- Stir in rice, reduce heat, cover pan and simmer for 20 minutes or until all liquid is absorbed.
- Fold cooked spinach into rice, add seasonings and serve hot.

*Or substitute one cup thawed frozen peas.

Veggie Pita Pizzas

Serves two

2 pita bread loaves
1 red or Vidalia onion, sliced
1 red bell pepper, sceded and
    sliced
¼ cup balsamic vinegar
¼ cup water
8 ounces mushrooms, sliced

olive oil cooking spray
4 tablespoons tomato sauce or
    fat-free Ragú® sauce
garlic powder to taste
¾ cup fat-free mozzarella
    cheese, grated

- Preheat oven to 325 degrees.
- Combine onion, red pepper, vinegar and water in a nonstick baking pan.
- Cover pan with aluminum foil and bake one hour and fifteen minutes or until vegetables are tender.
- Sauté mushrooms in a nonstick skillet sprayed with olive oil spray. Drain if needed.
- Place pita loaves on a sheet pan.
- Spread tomato sauce evenly on each pita loaf and sprinkle with garlic powder.
- Place onions, peppers and mushrooms evenly over loaves.
- Top pizzas with mozzarella cheese and bake in a 400 degree oven for about 15 minutes.
- Serve immediately with red pepper flakes, if desired.

Tossed Artichoke Heart and Tomato Salad with Creamy Chive Vinaigrette

Serves four

1½ tablespoons fat-free sour cream
1½ teaspoons Dijon mustard
1 tablespoon red wine vinegar with garlic
¼ teaspoon freshly squeezed lemon juice

1 tablespoon fresh chive, chopped
salt and freshly ground pepper to taste
4 cups mixed lettuce greens
6 artichoke hearts, quartered
1 large tomato, chopped
5 green onions, chopped (optional)

- Whisk together first five ingredients with salt and pepper.
- Place lettuce, artichoke hearts, tomato and green onions in a large bowl and toss with dressing.

You may substitute fat-free yogurt for fat-free sour cream in my recipes.

Fish and Corn Creole

Serves two to three

olive oil cooking spray
1 small onion, chopped
1 red bell pepper, chopped
2 cloves garlic, minced
1 14½-ounce can Italian style
    stewed tomatoes, un-
    drained and chopped
1 ear of corn, cooked, cut off
    the cob and puréed
1 ear of corn, cooked and cut
    off the cob
1 cup canned fat-free chicken broth

½ cup white wine
1 teaspoon Creole seasonings
    or to taste
salt and freshly ground pep-
    per to taste
¾ pound grouper fillet, cut in
    cubes
2 tablespoons fresh parsley,
    chopped
cooked rice
red hot sauce

- Spray a large nonstick deep skillet with cooking spray.
- Add onion and bell pepper and sauté until soft.
- Add next seven ingredients, salt and pepper and bring to a boil.
- Reduce heat and simmer 15 minutes.
- Add cubed grouper and cook until opaque, about 15 to 20 minutes.
- Add more white wine while fish is cooking if sauce becomes too thick.
- Spoon Fish and Corn Creole over cooked rice.
- Top with parsley and serve with red hot sauce on side.

Seafood Lasagna

Serves four

olive oil cooking spray
12 ounces fresh mushrooms,
    sliced
1 10-ounce package frozen
    chopped spinach, cooked
    and drained
¼ cup all-purpose flour
1¼ cup skim milk
¾ cup white wine
2 teaspoons minced garlic
1 tablespoon fat-free grated
    Parmesan cheese
salt to taste

pepper to taste
chili powder to taste
¾ pound scallops
6 no-boil lasagna noodles
8 ounces Louis Kemp®
    fat-free Crab Delights
3 tablespoons fresh basil,
    chopped
2 tablespoons fresh chive,
    chopped
1 cup fat-free mozzarella
    cheese, grated
paprika

- Preheat oven to 350 degrees.
- Sauté mushrooms in a pan sprayed with olive oil spray and set aside.
- Place flour in a saucepan and gradually add milk over a medium heat.
- Add ½ cup wine, garlic, Parmesan cheese, salt, pepper and chili powder and blend ingredients with a wire whisk.
- Cook for five minutes or until thickened.
- In a small saucepan, poach scallops in ¼ cup wine for about three minutes or until cooked through and opaque.
- Spoon a small amount of sauce in the bottom of an 8 x 8-inch baking pan sprayed with olive oil spray.
- Cover sauce with two dry lasagna noodles, side-by-side.
- Spoon spinach evenly over noodles. Season with salt and pepper.
- Cover spinach with two more lasagna noodles.
- Scatter scallops and crab over noodles and sprinkle with basil and additional salt and pepper.
- Top seafood with two more noodles and place mushrooms on top.
- Spoon remaining sauce evenly over all layers.

- Sprinkle top with chive, mozzarella cheese and paprika.
- Cover pan loosely with foil.
- Bake 30 minutes.
- Remove foil and bake an additional 15 minutes.
- Let stand ten minutes before cutting.

Making lasagna can be a tedious task if you are in a rush. This version is a breeze due to the creation of no-boil noodles. If you still find that this recipe is too time-intensive, broil a piece of fish, bake a potato, open a can of green beans. Remember, time limitations and laziness are no longer excuses for dashing to buy a grease-laden, high-fat, fast-food burger.

Vegetable Stew

Serves two as a main course

3 carrots, peeled and sliced diagonally
1 large onion, quartered
2 new potatoes, cut in half
1 turnip, peeled and cut in eighths
16 green beans, stringed
salt, pepper, garlic powder to taste

½ cup Healthy Choice® condensed cream of mushroom soup
½ cup water
½ cup Madeira wine
½ package dry onion soup mix
1 14½-ounce can of Italian style stewed tomatoes

Getting tired of my beloved zero-fat stewed tomatoes? If so, delete tomatoes and increase water to one cup.

- Preheat oven to 325 degrees.
- Place the carrots, onion, potatoes, turnip and green beans in a pot of rapidly boiling water for five minutes.
- Drain vegetables and place them in an ovenproof baking dish.
- Season vegetables with salt, pepper and garlic powder.
- In a small saucepan, over a low heat, mix together the mushroom soup, water, wine and dry onion soup mix and combine until the mixture is smooth.
- Pour the soup and wine mixture over the vegetables and top evenly with the tomatoes.
- Cover dish with aluminum foil and bake for at least one hour.
- Baking time will vary according to whether you prefer your vegetables tender or crisp. You may delete the parboiling step. If so, increase baking time.

Oven Grilled Vegetable Medley

Serves four

2 onions, peeled and cut into
    eighths
1 red bell pepper, halved,
    cored, seeded and cut in
    strips lengthwise

2 zucchini, cut in half horizon-
    tally and sliced in half or
    quartered lengthwise
¼ cup balsamic vinegar
¼ cup water
1 teaspoon minced garlic
salt and pepper to taste

- Preheat oven to 400 degrees.
- Place cut vegetables in a broiler-proof pan.
- Pour the vinegar and water over vegetables and toss with the garlic, salt and pepper.
- Cover pan with aluminum foil and bake vegetables for 45 minutes or until tender.
- Remove foil and place pan under the broiler for five minutes.

Reduce or increase cooking time according to your personal preference.

Cauliflower Au Gratin

Serves four to six

2 10-ounce packages frozen
    cauliflower, cooked and
    drained
1 15-ounce can Healthy
    Choice® cream of mush-
    room soup
¼ cup fat-free sour cream
1 tablespoon Dijon mustard

¾ cup fat-free cheddar cheese,
    grated
¼ cup fat-free Parmesan
    cheese
salt and pepper to taste
¼ cup Italian style bread
    crumbs
olive oil cooking spray

- Preheat oven to 350 degrees.
- Lightly spray a 1½-quart casserole with cooking spray.
- Place cauliflower, seasoned with salt and pepper, in the casserole dish.
- Stir together the soup, sour cream, mustard and cheeses in a medium saucepan.
- Heat the soup mixture until the ingredients are well-combined.
- Pour the sauce over the cauliflower.
- Sprinkle the bread crumbs over the sauce.
- Bake uncovered for 35 to 40 minutes or until bubbling.

One and a half pounds steamed broccoli is a wonderful alternative to cauliflower in this recipe.

Sweet and Sour Glazed Carrots

Serves four

16 baby carrots, peeled
salt
1 tablespoon balsamic vinegar

1½ tablespoons brown sugar
chopped parsley

- In a saucepan, cook carrots in water* with salt until tender.
- Transfer drained carrots to a medium nonstick skillet.
- Add vinegar and brown sugar and stir carrots over a medium heat until vinegar evaporates and sugar melts.
- Garnish with chopped parsley.

*or fat-free chicken broth

Had a hard day and want a quick and delicious Chinese dinner? Steam a few broccoli crowns and sugar snap peas. Sauté some sliced mushrooms in olive oil cooking spray. Spray a wok or deep skillet with olive oil cooking spray. Stir-fry a couple of coarsely chopped celery sticks with one small chopped onion. Add one boneless, skinless cubed chicken breast, seasoned with salt and pepper and sauté until chicken is almost cooked. Whisk together a liquid mixture comprised of at least one cup fat-free chicken broth, two teaspoons lite soy sauce and one heaping table-spoon cornstarch. Add liquid mixture to chicken and cook over low heat until sauce thickens. Stir in broccoli, peapods, mushrooms and a few sliced water chestnuts and bamboo shoots. Add some minced garlic and a few dashes of Worcestershire sauce. Adjust soy flavoring, salt and pepper and serve hot over rice. *Serves two.*

Tossing in a few peeled shrimp makes a great addition to this dish. Remember: creative cooking means putting your own signature on my recipes.

Turkey Stroganoff

Serves four

olive oil cooking spray
1 onion, chopped
1 celery stick, chopped
1 pound ground turkey breast
1½ teaspoons minced garlic
salt and pepper to taste
1 15-ounce can Healthy
    Choice® cream of mush-
    room soup
⅔ cup chicken broth
½ cup white wine

1 8-ounce can sliced mush-
    rooms, drained
1 cup frozen peas, thawed
2 tablespoons tomato paste
1 tablespoon Worcestershire
    sauce or to taste
2 tablespoons fat-free sour
    cream
12 ounces yolk-free noodles,
    cooked
fat-free grated Parmesan
    cheese

- Sauté onions and celery until soft in a nonstick skillet sprayed with olive oil spray.
- Add crumbled ground turkey, garlic and salt and pepper and cook until turkey is done.
- In a saucepan, stir together soup, broth, wine, mushrooms, and bring mixture to a boil. Reduce heat and simmer ten minutes.
- Pour soup mixture into skillet with turkey.
- Stir in peas, tomato paste and Worcestershire sauce.
- Simmer Stroganoff for 30 minutes.
- Add sour cream, adjust seasonings and continue to simmer for an additional 15 minutes.
- Serve over noodles with Parmesan cheese.

Several splashes of Madeira wine and a couple shakes of chili powder add zip to this Stroganoff.

Artichoke, Tomato and Corn Salad

Serves two as main course
Serves four as side dish

1 artichoke bottom, coarsely
chopped
1 14-ounce can artichoke
hearts, drained and quar-
tered
2 tomatoes, chopped
2 ears of corn, cooked and cut
off the cob
1 bunch green onions,
chopped

2 tablespoons fresh basil,
chopped
1 tablespoon fresh chive,
chopped
2 tablespoons balsamic
vinegar
salt and pepper to taste
1 artichoke, steamed and
chilled

- Mix together first eight ingredients and season with salt and pep-
per.
- Place the salad mixture in the center of each plate.
- Surround the salad mixture with the artichoke leaves and serve.

To cook a whole artichoke:

- Trim artichoke stem.
- Cut off about one inch of top.
- Snip prickly tips of artichoke with scissors.
- Place artichoke in pan of boiling water and boil gently until
leaves pull away easily (anywhere from 40-60 minutes).

To prepare artichoke bottom:

- Remove leaves of cooked artichoke until you reach the hairy
choke.
- Scrape away the choke with a small knife or teaspoon until
the bottom is revealed and all the "hair" is removed.

Eggplant Parmigiana

Serves four

olive oil cooking spray
1 peeled eggplant, cut into
  one-half inch slices
½ cup Italian style bread
  crumbs
1 cup fat-free ricotta cheese
½ cup fat-free grated Parmesan cheese

1 teaspoon oregano
1 teaspoon minced garlic
salt and pepper to taste
2 cups Ragú® fat-free tomato
  pasta sauce
1½ cups fat-free grated mozzarella cheese

- Preheat broiler.
- Spray olive oil spray on a baking sheet.
- Put bread crumbs in a shallow bowl.
- Lightly spray each cut side of eggplant with cooking spray and coat each side with bread crumbs.
- Place eggplant on baking sheet and broil for four minutes per side or until slightly browned.
- Spray an 8 x 8-inch baking pan with cooking spray and place half the eggplant slices in one overlapping layer.
- Mix together the ricotta cheese, Parmesan cheese, oregano, garlic, salt and pepper in a bowl.
- Spoon the ricotta cheese mixture on top of the eggplant.
- Pour half the tomato sauce over the ricotta cheese.
- Place another layer of eggplant over the sauce.
- Pour remaining sauce evenly over casserole and top with grated mozzarella cheese.
- Cover dish with foil and bake in a preheated 350 degree oven for 30 minutes.
- Uncover and bake for an additional 15 minutes.
- Let eggplant rest for a few minutes before slicing into squares.

Experience a great taste sensation by adding a middle layer of grilled portobello mushrooms.

Maple-Dijon Barbecue Chicken

Serves two

2 boneless chicken breast
 halves, skinned
2 tablespoons pure maple
 syrup

3 tablespoons bottled chili
 sauce
1 tablespoon cider vinegar
1 tablespoon Dijon mustard
salt and pepper to taste

- Preheat oven to 350 degrees.
- Season chicken with salt and pepper.
- Place chicken in a small nonmetallic baking pan.
- To make sauce: combine syrup, chili sauce, vinegar and mustard in a small saucepan and stir together over a low heat for a few minutes.
- Pour sauce over chicken and add a small amount of water to the bottom of the pan.
- Bake for about 25 minutes or until chicken is tender.

This Maple-Dijon Barbecue Sauce is wonderful with pork tenderloin. Prepare your grill to medium-high heat or preheat broiler. Grill pork eight minutes per side. Serve warm sauce on the side.

Tomato and Corn Salsa

Serves two

1 large tomato, peeled and
    chopped coarsely
1 cup fresh cooked or canned
    corn
2 tablespoons red onion,
    chopped

1 tablespoon cilantro,
    chopped or 1 tablespoon
    basil, chopped
1½ tablespoons red wine vine-
    gar with garlic
salt and freshly ground pep-
    per to taste

- Stir together all ingredients in a bowl and serve.

Also delicious with one cup drained and rinsed canned black beans and chopped green chili peppers to taste.

Tired of your own kitchen? Take a break and go out to dinner if you promise to keep two provisos in mind. Condition number one: do not leave *The Paty Plan* principles at home. Condition number two: *Lie!* Order a piece of chicken or fish, a baked potato and a salad with balsamic vinegar. Then be sure to tell your waiter you are allergic to butter and oil. If not, the chef will prepare your dishes with two of *The Paty Plan* big "don'ts." Don't let that happen!

Italian Vegetable Stew

Serves two

olive oil cooking spray
1 onion, chopped
1 red pepper, chopped
1 zucchini, chopped
1 cup fat-free chicken broth
1 15.5-ounce can cannellini
    beans, drained
1 14.5-ounce can Italian style
    stewed tomatoes

1 cup fat-free Ragú® tomato
    and basil sauce
2 teaspoons minced garlic
1 teaspoon dried oregano
salt, pepper and chili powder
    to taste
6 ounces fresh spinach
fat-free Parmesan cheese
fat-free mozzarella cheese

- Sauté onion and red pepper until almost soft in a deep nonstick skillet sprayed with olive oil cooking spray.
- Stir in zucchini and continue to sauté for a couple of minutes.
- Add chicken broth and bring to a boil.
- Reduce heat and simmer five minutes.
- Add next five ingredients plus salt, pepper and chili powder.
- Return mixture to a boil.
- Reduce heat and simmer for fifteen minutes.
- While mixture is simmering, sauté spinach in a nonstick skillet sprayed with olive oil cooking spray.
- Add spinach to stew immediately before serving and adjust seasonings.
- Top stew with mixture of cheeses.

Zippy Italian Lima Beans

Serves four

1 10-ounce package frozen
    lima beans, cooked
1 14½-ounce can Italian style
    stewed tomatoes,
    chopped

½ teaspoon dried oregano
1 teaspoon prepared horse-
    radish or to taste
salt and pepper

- Combine all ingredients in a saucepan and cook over a medium heat until hot.

Stir in a can of Italian style stewed tomatoes to cooked green beans, okra or zucchini for a nutritious vegetable dish.

On a low cholesterol diet? Prepare this "creamy" shrimpless corn chowder: Sauté one small finely chopped onion and one finely chopped red pepper until soft in a nonstick saucepan sprayed with olive oil cooking spray. Add two cups fat-free chicken broth and bring to a boil. Reduce heat and simmer for 15 minutes. Add one 15.25-ounce can corn or three ears cooked corn cut off the cob and one 15.25 ounce can cream-style corn. Whisk together one teaspoon Wondra® quick mixing flour with ¾ cup skim milk. Stir the milk mixture into the saucepan. Add ¼ cup Madeira wine, one heaping teaspoon canned chopped green chilies, one tablespoon instant mashed potatoes, salt, pepper and a dash of chili powder. Continue to simmer for 15 minutes. Serve hot with chopped fresh chive. *Serves three.*

Shrimp and Corn Chowder

Serves four

olive oil cooking spray
1 medium onion, chopped
3 cups fat-free chicken broth
2 medium potatoes, peeled
  and chopped
2 cups fresh corn, cooked and
  cut off the cob
1 8½-ounce can cream style
  corn
½ cup white wine

½ cup cold skim milk
1 tablespoon Wondra® quick
  mixing flour
⅓ cup cilantro, chopped
1 pound uncooked shrimp,
  peeled
⅛ teaspoon chili powder
salt and freshly ground pepper to taste
fresh chive, chopped

- Sauté onion until soft in a deep nonstick skillet sprayed with olive oil cooking spray.
- Add chicken broth and potatoes and cook until potatoes are tender.
- Add fresh corn, cream-style corn and white wine and stir over a medium-low heat.
- Mix together milk and flour and stir into the corn mixture.
- Add seasonings, cilantro, shrimp and cook for about three minutes or until shrimp is done.
- Serve chowder garnished with chive.

Tomato Bruschetta

Serves four

3 tomatoes, peeled, seeded
    and chopped
½ cup fresh basil, chopped
2 garlic cloves, peeled and
    minced
1 teaspoon balsamic vinegar

salt and freshly ground pep-
    per to taste
4 ¾-inch slices Italian bread or
    French baguette
2 garlic cloves, peeled and
    halved lengthwise

- Preheat broiler.
- Toss together first four ingredients and season with salt and pepper.
- Place bread on broiler rack and broil on both sides until golden brown.
- Remove the bread and rub each side with the cut side of the garlic halves.
- Mount tomato mixture on top of bread slices and serve.

Never refrigerate tomatoes as they will lose their marvelous flavor.

To peel and seed tomatoes: place tomatoes in a pan of boiling water for 30 seconds. Drain the tomatoes in a colander and run cold water over them. The skin will easily peel away with a knife after they have cooled. Cut the peeled tomatoes in half and squeeze each half gently to expel the seeds.

Broccoli Cheese Squares

Serves six

olive oil cooking spray
2 10-ounce packages frozen
    chopped broccoli, cooked
    and drained
1 onion, chopped
1 teaspoon garlic, minced
1 cup Egg Beaters®

¼ cup skim milk
⅓ cup Italian style bread
    crumbs
1 cup fat-free cheddar cheese,
    grated
salt and freshly ground pep-
    per to taste

- Preheat oven to 350 degrees.
- Combine broccoli, onion and garlic in a bowl.
- In a separate bowl, combine eggs and milk.
- Combine broccoli mixture with egg mixture.
- Add remaining ingredients and spoon into an 8 x 8-inch nonstick baking pan sprayed with cooking spray.
- Bake 35 to 40 minutes or until set.
- Cool slightly and cut into squares.

Scalloped Potatoes

Serves four to six

2 large potatoes, peeled and
thinly sliced
1 large onion, chopped
1¼ cups fat-free mozzarella
cheese
olive oil cooking spray
generous amounts of salt,
pepper and garlic powder

1 cup Egg Beaters®
1 cup skim milk
¼ cup fat-free Parmesan
cheese
paprika

- Preheat oven to 350 degrees.
- Place one-third of the sliced potatoes in an 8 x 8-inch nonstick baking pan sprayed generously with cooking spray.
- Season potatoes with salt, pepper and garlic powder.
- Sprinkle one-third of the onions over the potatoes.
- Sprinkle one-third of the mozzarella cheese over the onions.
- Repeat layers ending with cheese.
- Whisk together the Egg Beaters® and milk.
- Pour egg mixture evenly over potatoes.
- Cover pan loosely with aluminum foil.
- Bake for one hour.
- After one hour, remove foil and top potatoes with Parmesan cheese and paprika.
- Bake an additional 15 minutes or until potatoes are tender.
- Cool slightly and cut into squares.

For the hungry chef in a hurry: heat together one 27½-ounce jar Ragú® fat-free pasta sauce with one 14½-ounce can stewed tomatoes and one 8-ounce can sliced mushrooms. Toss with your favorite cooked pasta. *Serves four.*

Creamy Italian Baked Ziti

Serves four

olive oil cooking spray
1 onion, chopped
1 pound ground turkey breast
salt and pepper
2 teaspoons minced garlic
1 14½-ounce can Italian style
    stewed tomatoes
1 16-ounce can tomato sauce
½ cup red wine
3 ounces tomato paste
¼ teaspoon chili powder
1 teaspoon dried oregano

1½ packages Equal® or to
    taste
½ cup fresh basil, chopped
½ cup cold skim milk
2 teaspoons Wondra® quick-
    mixing flour
8 ounces dried ziti
½ cup fat-free grated Parme-
    san cheese
1¼ cups fat-free mozzarella
    cheese, grated

- Sauté onion until soft in a large deep skillet sprayed with cooking spray.
- Add turkey, salt, pepper and garlic and cook until turkey is done.
- Stir in tomatoes, tomato sauce, wine and tomato paste.
- In a bowl, whisk together milk and Wondra® quick-mixing flour.
- Stir the milk mixture into the turkey-tomato mixture.
- Adjust seasonings and simmer sauce for one hour.
- Meanwhile, cook pasta in a pot of boiling water until done but firm to the bite.
- Stir pasta into sauce and mix in Parmesan cheese.
- Place pasta and sauce mixture in a casserole dish and cover loosely with aluminum foil.
- Bake covered casserole in a preheated 350 degree oven for 30 minutes.
- Uncover casserole and top with mozzarella cheese.
- Bake uncovered for an additional 15 minutes.

German Fried Potatoes

Serves two

olive oil cooking spray
2 baked potatoes, cooled and
cut into ½-inch slices

salt, pepper, garlic powder
and paprika

- Spray a large nonstick skillet with cooking spray.
- Place the potato slices in the skillet and season liberally with salt, pepper, garlic powder and paprika.
- Cook the potatoes over a medium-high heat until brown on one side.
- Turn potatoes, season and brown well on the other side. Serve hot.

I love these served with a dollop of ketchup.

Cajun New Potatoes

Serves four

olive oil cooking spray
16 small new potatoes, un-
    peeled, or 8 large new po-
    tatoes, unpeeled and
    halved

¼ cup Dijon mustard
1¼ teaspoons Creole season-
    ing
salt, freshly ground pepper
    and garlic powder

- Preheat oven to 375 degrees.
- Boil potatoes in salted water until tender.
- Place drained potatoes in a nonstick roasting pan generously sprayed with cooking spray.
- Spoon the mustard evenly over potatoes.
- Sprinkle potatoes with Creole seasoning and toss with liberal amounts of other seasonings.
- Bake for 45 minutes.

You may want to spray potatoes with olive oil cooking spray while potatoes are roasting.

Turkey Burger

Serves two

olive oil cooking spray
12 ounces ground turkey
salt and pepper

garlic powder
Worcestershire sauce
lite soy sauce

- Spray a nonstick skillet with cooking spray.
- Divide ground turkey in half and shape into two equal burgers.
- Place burgers in skillet and sprinkle top side with seasonings.
- Shake liberal amounts of Worcestershire and soy sauce over turkey.
- Sear over high heat for about four minutes.
- Turn burger, sprinkle more seasonings and sauces, and sear for an additional four minutes.
- Lower heat to low-medium and continue to cook an additional five minutes per side or until cooked through.
- Serve with mustard or ketchup.

My husband and I adore ground turkey but cheaper is not better. I purchase Perdue® ground turkey products.

Uncreamed Onions

Serves two

2 red onions, peeled   ¼ cup red wine
¼ cup balsamic vinegar   ¼ cup water

- Preheat oven to 350 degrees.
- Cut onions in half and quarter each half.
- Place onions in a nonstick baking pan.
- Pour vinegar, wine and water over onions.
- Cover pan with aluminum foil.
- Bake for at least one hour or until tender.

Use Sweet Vidalia or Walla Walla onions when in season.

Another quick and easy onion idea: peel one Vidalia or Walla Walla onion. Scoop out a hole in the center. Place onion in a baking dish. Pour one-half cup fat-free chicken broth over onion. Fill center with a heaping tablespoon of prepared mango chutney. Cover pan with aluminum foil and bake in a preheated 350 degree oven for one hour or until tender.

Tuna and Pasta Salad

Serves four

4 ounces dried rotelle pasta, cooked according to package directions and drained

1 6 ⅛-ounce can tuna in water, drained

1 15½-ounce can garbanzo beans, drained and rinsed

3 tablespoons red onion, chopped

1 tomato, chopped

⅓ cup fresh basil, chopped

salt and generous amounts of cracked pepper

- Combine all ingredients in a bowl.

Dressing . . .

¼ teaspoon anchovy paste

½ cup red wine vinegar

1 tablespoon Dijon mustard

½ teaspoon minced garlic

- Whisk together dressing ingredients.
- Add dressing to salad and toss.

Not flavorful enough for you? Toss in a little of my Quick and Easy Italian Dressing* or your favorite fat-free salad dressing. Do the same with my rice salad recipes.

Rice and Spinach Stuffed Tomatoes

Serves six

6 tomatoes
1 package long grain and wild
    rice, cooked according to
    package directions
1 10-ounce package frozen
    chopped spinach, cooked
    and drained

6 spring onions, chopped
¾ cup fat-free mozzarella
    cheese, grated
½ cup fat-free grated Parme-
    san cheese
salt and pepper
olive oil cooking spray

- Slice off top of each tomato and scoop out insides leaving a firm shell.
- Chop tomato pulp.
- Invert tomatoes and drain.
- Combine pulp with the next six ingredients.
- Spoon rice mixture into tomatoes.
- Spray tops of tomatoes lightly with cooking spray.
- Bake uncovered in a preheated 350 degree oven for 20 minutes.

Leftover rice mixture is great reheated in microwave.

Turkey Enchilada Casserole

Serves four

olive oil cooking spray
1 onion, chopped
1 pound ground turkey breast
¼ teaspoon chili powder or to taste
½ teaspoon ground cumin or to taste
salt and pepper to taste
1 15-ounce can black beans, rinsed and drained

1 8.5-ounce can corn
1 cup chunky salsa
¾ cup fat-free mozzarella cheese, grated
8 6-inch corn tortillas
1 14.5-ounce can Mexican style stewed tomatoes
1 cup fat-free cheddar cheese, grated

- Preheat oven to 350 degrees.
- Spray an 8" x 8" deep baking pan with olive oil spray.
- Spray a large skillet with olive oil spray and sauté onions until tender.
- Add ground turkey and seasonings to onion and brown until turkey is fully cooked.
- Stir in the beans, corn and salsa and simmer mixture for five minutes.
- Overlap four tortillas on bottom of the baking pan, covering completely.
- Spoon half of the turkey mixture evenly over the tortillas.
- Sprinkle the mozzarella cheese evenly over the turkey mixture.
- Cover with remaining four tortillas.
- Spoon remaining turkey mixture over tortillas.
- Pour tomatoes with their juices evenly over the turkey mixture.
- Cover pan with aluminum foil.
- Bake casserole for 35 minutes.
- Remove foil and top casserole with cheddar cheese.
- Continue to bake uncovered for an additional 15 minutes or until bubbling.
- Let stand ten minutes before cutting.

To roast and mash garlic: put unpeeled garlic cloves loosely in aluminum foil and place in a 350 degree preheated oven for 30 minutes. Remove from oven and squeeze garlic out of its skin. Place in a small bowl and mash with tines of a fork.

Garlic Mashed Potatoes

Serves two as a main course
Serves four as a side dish

4 potatoes, peeled and quartered

2 cups fat-free chicken broth or turkey broth

water

1 cup skim milk

1 cup fat-free cheddar cheese, grated (optional)

3 cloves roasted garlic, mashed or garlic powder to taste

salt and freshly ground pepper

- Place potatoes in a large saucepan and cover with salted broth and water.
- Bring potatoes to a boil.
- Reduce heat and simmer until potatoes are tender.
- Drain potatoes and transfer to a large bowl.
- Mash potatoes with a potato masher or electric mixer until smooth. While mashing, slowly add skim milk.
- Return potatoes to the saucepan and place under a low heat.
- Add cheese, garlic, salt and pepper and stir vigorously until hot.
- Serve immediately.

Reduce skim milk to ½ cup and add ½ cup fat-free chicken broth for a slightly different taste.

Mushroom Stuffed Pasta Shells

Serves four

olive oil cooking spray
8 ounces fresh mushrooms,
    chopped finely by hand
    or in a food processor
1 15-ounce container fat-free
    ricotta cheese
¼ cup fat-free Parmesan
    cheese
2 teaspoons minced garlic
1 teaspoon dried oregano

2 tablespoons fresh basil,
    chopped
salt and pepper to taste
3 cups prepared fat-free to-
    mato pasta sauce
16 jumbo pasta shells, cooked
    according to package di-
    rections
1 cup fat-free mozzarella
    cheese, grated

- Preheat oven to 375 degrees.
- Sauté mushrooms in a small skillet sprayed with cooking spray.
- In a mixing bowl, stir together the mushrooms with the next five ingredients. Season with salt and pepper.
- Pour one cup of the tomato pasta sauce in the bottom of a baking dish.
- Spoon the mushroom mixture into the pasta shells and place on top of the sauce.
- Pour the remaining sauce over the shells and top with the mozzarella cheese.
- Bake for 30 minutes or until bubbly.

Grits with Shrimp Sauce

Serves four

olive oil cooking spray
2 shallots, chopped
1 small onion, chopped finely
2 celery stalks, chopped finely
1½ teaspoons minced garlic
2 cups fat-free chicken broth
1 14½-ounce can Italian style
    stewed tomatoes
½ cup white wine
⅛ teaspoon chili powder
20 fresh shrimp, peeled

salt and freshly ground pepper
4 servings grits, cooked ac-
    cording to package direc-
    tions with salt and white
    pepper to taste
2 ears of corn, cooked and cut
    off the cob
⅓ cup fat-free grated Parme-
    san cheese
fresh chive, chopped

- Spray a large nonstick skillet with cooking spray.
- Add shallots, onion, celery and sauté until soft.
- Add garlic, stock, tomatoes, wine and seasonings and bring to a boil.
- Reduce heat to medium-low and simmer mixture for 25 minutes.
- Add shrimp and cook for an additional two to three minutes or until shrimp is done and adjust seasonings.
- While shrimp is cooking, stir together hot cooked grits, corn and Parmesan cheese and heat until cheese is melted.
- Serve shrimp sauce over grits in pasta bowls and top with fresh chive.

My Southern friends would be horrified, but I adore my grits extra thick and "mashed" with this shrimp recipe. For "mashed grits": stir in ½ tablespoon instant potatoes and ¼ cup skim milk to seasoned grits during last minutes of cooking. Add corn, Parmesan cheese and serve hot topped with shrimp sauce and chive.

Go ahead and treat yourself to pork tenderloin in place of chicken one night. The best recipes are the simplest.

Season 1½ pounds pork tenderloin with salt, pepper and minced garlic or garlic powder. Broil or grill tenderloin for eight to ten minutes per side or until done. *Serves four.*

Or

To create a succulent version: mix together one cup prepared chunky salsa and two tablespoons apricot preserves. Spoon sauce evenly over 1½ pounds pork tenderloin and cook in a 375 degree preheated oven for 35 minutes or until cooked through. Serve with cabbage braised in fat-free chicken stock and steamed sugar snap pea pods. *Serves four.*

Georgia-Mex Chicken

Serves four

4 chicken breast halves, 	1 cup prepared chunky salsa
   skinned and boned 	2 tablespoons peach preserves

- Preheat oven to 350 degrees.
- Place chicken breasts in a baking pan.
- In a small bowl, mix together the salsa and peach preserves.
- Spoon the Georgia-Mex sauce evenly over the chicken.
- Bake chicken for 30 to 35 minutes or until done.

Chicken Supreme

Serves four

4 chicken breasts, skinned and
  boned
olive oil cooking spray
salt and pepper to taste
1 teaspoon minced garlic
12 ounces fresh mushrooms,
  sliced

1 15-ounce can Healthy
  Choice® cream of mush-
  room soup
⅓ cup white wine
2 tablespoons fat-free sour
  cream
1 teaspoon tomato paste
¼ cup fat-free grated Parmesan cheese

- Preheat oven to 350 degrees.
- Season chicken with salt and pepper.
- Brown chicken on each side with garlic in a deep nonstick skillet sprayed with olive oil spray. Do not burn garlic.
- Place chicken in a baking dish.
- Sauté mushrooms in the same skillet sprayed with additional olive oil spray.
- Add remaining ingredients to mushrooms and heat until mixture is well-combined.
- Pour sauce over chicken and bake for 30 minutes or until done.
- Serve chicken and sauce with rice.

Serve the Chicken Supreme* with my Rice and Spinach Stuffed Tomatoes* for a colorful wintertime repast. Prepare the Chicken and Wild Rice Salad* stuffed in fresh tomatoes for a cooler alternative during the summer months.

Another beautiful summer shrimp salad supper:

4 cups mixed salad
   greens
2 new potatoes, boiled,
   chilled and sliced
16 green beans, steamed
   and chilled
1 large tomato, chopped
   or 1 small red
   pepper, chopped

1 ear of corn, cooked
   and cut off the cob
16 fresh shrimp, boiled,
   peeled and chilled
3 green onions, chopped
fresh chive, chopped

Assemble all ingredients on two dinner plates. Serve
with Quick and Easy Italian Dressing.*

Won the lottery or just received a big income tax refund?
Add some lobster meat!

Summer Salmon and Shrimp

Serves two

2 tomatoes, chopped
1 small cucumber, chopped
1 yellow bell pepper, chopped
2 tablespoons finely chopped
    red onion
1 tablespoon fresh basil,
    chopped
2 tablespoons balsamic vine-
    gar

salt and pepper to taste
2 6-ounce pink salmon fillets,
    grilled, broiled or
    poached (about six min-
    utes per side) and chilled
12 shrimp, boiled, peeled and
    chilled
1 tablespoon capers

- Mix together first six ingredients and season with salt and pepper.
- Divide tomato mixture and place on individual plates.
- Top tomato mixture with a salmon fillet.
- Top salmon fillets with shrimp and capers.
- Serve poolside or anywhere!

Chicken and Wild Rice Salad

Serves six

3½ cups degreased homemade chicken stock or fat-free canned chicken broth
1 6-ounce package long grain and wild rice with seasonings
½ cup white rice
4 skinned, boned and seasoned chicken breast halves, grilled, broiled or baked and diced
1¼ cups frozen peas, thawed
1 bunch green onions, peeled and chopped
¼ cup fresh basil, chopped or 2 teaspoons fresh tarragon
salt and pepper to taste

Dressing:
⅓ cup red wine vinegar
1 tablespoon Dijon mustard
2 teaspoons garlic, minced
1 tablespoon fat-free sour cream

- Bring the chicken stock to a boil in a medium saucepan.
- Stir in long grain and wild rice with seasonings and white rice to boiling stock.
- Cover pan tightly, reduce heat and simmer for 20 minutes or until all the liquid is absorbed.
- Cool cooked rice and place in a large bowl.
- Add the chicken, peas, onion and basil to the rice. Season with salt and pepper.
- In a separate bowl, whisk together dressing ingredients.
- Toss the chicken and rice mixture with the dressing and adjust seasonings.
- Serve salad on a bed of your favorite lettuce.

You will have a beautiful presentation if you stuff this salad into fresh tomatoes.

115

Corn, Rice and Black Bean Salad

Serves four

2 cups cooked rice
2 ears of corn, cooked and cut
    off the cob
1 15-ounce can black beans,
    rinsed and drained
3 tablespoons red onion,
    chopped

3 tablespoons fresh basil,
    shredded
chili powder, salt and pepper
    to taste
1 ounce red wine vinegar with
    garlic or balsamic vinegar

- Mix together first six ingredients, add seasonings and chill.
- Thirty minutes before serving, remove salad from refrigerator and toss with vinegar.

This salad is a delicious accompaniment to Grilled Pork Tenderloin.

Turkey, Barley, Vegetable Soup

Serves six

2 cups leftover cooked turkey breast meat, cubed
1 turkey breast carcass
10 cups water
1 large onion, coarsely chopped
3 stalks celery, coarsely chopped
2 bay leaves

½ pound fresh green beans, stringed and snapped in thirds
1 14½-ounce can stewed tomatoes
1½ cups fresh carrots, diced
1 cup frozen lima beans
salt, pepper, dried oregano, and chili powder or your favorite seasonings
½ cup barley

- Place cubed turkey meat and carcass with bone in a large soup pot.
- Add the water, onion, celery and bay leaves. Bring the pot to a boil.
- Lower the heat and simmer for two hours with the pot partially covered. Skim any froth that rises to the top.
- Remove and slightly cool the carcass. Return any turkey meat from the carcass to the pot.
- Add green beans, tomatoes and seasonings. Return the pot to a boil.
- Reduce heat and simmer partially-covered for 30 minutes.
- Add carrots and lima beans and simmer for an additional 40 minutes.
- Add barley and continue to simmer for another 30 minutes or until barley is done.
- Adjust seasonings and serve after bay leaves are removed.

While preparing this recipe, add water during the simmering process if the soup becomes too thick. The cooled soup freezes beautifully and can be pulled out on a cold winter night.

Cooking is not an exact science. I am constantly changing and revising my own recipes. Please let your creative juices flow when you prepare my dishes. Add more seasonings, adjust wine or broth amounts. Just be sure not to improvise with added fat grams.

Mushroom-Barley Risotto

Serves four

olive oil cooking spray
12 white mushrooms, chopped
6 ounces portobello mushrooms, chopped
1 onion, chopped
1½ cups medium barley
6 cups fat-free chicken broth
¼ cup Madeira wine
1 tablespoon minced garlic
2 tablespoons tomato paste
¼ cup fat-free Parmesan cheese
salt and pepper to taste
6 green onions, chopped

- Sauté white mushrooms and portobello mushrooms in a pan sprayed with olive oil cooking spray and set aside.
- Sauté chopped onions in a deep nonstick saucepan sprayed with cooking spray until slightly browned.
- Stir in the barley.
- Add four cups chicken broth to the onions and barley and bring to a boil.
- Reduce heat to low and cover pan.
- Cook for 30 minutes and add more broth if liquid is absorbing too quickly.
- Stir occasionally.
- Stir in mushrooms, Madeira wine, minced garlic, tomato paste, salt and pepper.
- Remove cover and continue to simmer for another 30 minutes or until barley is tender. Add more broth if needed while simmering.
- While barley is cooking, sauté green onions in olive oil cooking spray until slightly browned.
- Stir Parmesan cheese into cooked barley.
- Adjust seasonings and serve in pasta bowls.
- Top Mushroom-Barley Risotto with browned onions.

Poached Fish Rossa with New Potatoes

Serves two

2 8-ounce pieces of orange
    roughy
2 new potatoes, boiled and
    sliced
salt and pepper
olive oil cooking spray
2 shallots, chopped

1 medium onion, sliced
1 14½-ounce can Italian style
    stewed tomatoes
1 cup white wine
1 teaspoon minced garlic
chili powder to taste

- Preheat oven to 375 degrees.
- Place fish in baking dish.
- Place potato slices along the outer sides of each fish piece and season with salt and pepper.
- Spray a nonstick deep skillet with olive oil cooking spray and sauté the shallots and onion slices until soft. Do not brown.
- Add the tomatoes, wine, garlic, chili powder, salt and pepper. Bring mixture to a boil.
- Reduce heat and simmer 15 minutes.
- Pour the tomato mixture evenly over the fish and potatoes and cover baking dish with foil.
- Bake for about 20 to 25 minutes or until fish is done.

Great Northern Bean and Spinach Gratin

Serves six

1 pound Great Northern beans, rinsed, sorted and soaked
2 onions, peeled and chopped
1 quart homemade or canned fat-free chicken stock
2 cups water
12 ounces fresh spinach, washed and dried
olive oil cooking spray

1 14½-ounce can Italian style stewed tomatoes, drained and chopped
2 heaping teaspoons minced garlic, divided
¾ to 1 teaspoon dried oregano or to taste
salt and coarsely ground pepper

- Place beans in a large pot and add the onion, chicken stock and water.
- Bring beans to a boil and reduce heat. Simmer partially covered for 1½ to 2 hours or until tender.
- Sauté the spinach in a pan sprayed with cooking spray.
- Drain the cooked beans in a colander placed over a bowl.
- Return the "pot likker" to the pan and boil for ten minutes or until reduced to one cup.
- Purée in a blender one cup of the beans, the reduced "likker" and one teaspoon garlic.
- Mix together the beans with the puréed mixture, spinach, tomatoes, remaining garlic, oregano and season with salt and pepper to taste.
- Spoon the mixture into a 3-quart casserole dish and bake in a 350 degree preheated oven for 40 minutes or until hot and bubbly.

Is it a poultry night? Spoon Great Northern Bean and Spinach Gratin into pasta bowls and top each serving with two pieces of cooked, drained and crumbled turkey bacon.

I always quick soak my beans. To do so: in a large pot, combine the beans with six cups of water. Bring to a boil and boil for two minutes. Remove from heat, cover pan and let beans stand for one hour. Drain and cook according to package or recipe directions.

Simply do not have the time or inclination to soak and cook dried beans? Do not be distressed. You will be the beneficiary of good (not great) nutrition and flavor if you open, drain, mix and heat together:

1 can navy beans   salt, pepper, garlic and
1 can stewed tomatoes   oregano to taste
1 can spinach

Remember, time excuses are not forgivable.

Seafood Florentine

Serves four

1 cup rice, cooked according
   to package directions and
   seasoned with salt and
   pepper
olive oil cooking spray
12 ounces fresh spinach,
   washed and dried
¼ cup flour
1 cup skim milk

½ cup dry vermouth
1 4½-ounce can shrimp, partially drained
¼ cup plus 1 tablespoon
   fat-free Parmesan cheese
4 6-ounce flounder or orange
   roughy fillets
salt and pepper
paprika

- Preheat oven to 350 degrees.
- Spray a large nonstick skillet with cooking spray and sauté spin-
  ach until wilted.
- Place flour in a saucepan and gradually add milk over a medium
  heat.
- Add wine, shrimp, ¼ cup Parmesan cheese. Season with salt and
  pepper to taste.
- Stir together ingredients for about five minutes or until thick-
  ened.
- Place the rice in the bottom of a broiler-proof baking dish
  sprayed with olive oil cooking spray and top with spinach.
- Place the fish fillets over the spinach and sprinkle with salt and
  pepper.
- Pour the sauce over the fish and cover pan with aluminum foil.
- Bake for 15 minutes. Remove foil, sprinkle the casserole with ad-
  ditional Parmesan cheese and paprika.
- Continue to bake uncovered for another ten minutes.
- Remove the dish from the oven and place in the broiler.
- Broil for five minutes or until top is lightly browned and fish is
  done.

The "I hate to cook!" or "I'm too busy to cook!" Syndrome

Syndrome Number One—"I hate to cook!"

On a recent trip to my parents in Naples, Florida, our family invited my aunt and cousin to dinner after their lengthy drive from the New England coast to the southern Gulf Shore. After dinner I showed my cousin *The Paty Plan* manuscript. As she was looking it over, she repeatedly said, "I hate to cook!" My husband and I stopped counting her repetitive exclamation after about the tenth time. We had gotten her message. Even the simplest of recipes in my book might not lend themselves to one who "hates to cook!"

Syndrome Number Two—"I'm too busy to cook!"

This syndrome hit me in the head at a party celebrating a friend's birthday. Someone was chatting about the need to lose weight before a beach vacation. She had heard of *The Paty Plan*, but it was her understanding that it would not work for her because she was "too busy to cook!" My normally steady blood pressure rose and I fumed all the way home. In my opinion, people might not like to cook, but few people are "too busy to cook!" If one has time to drive to a fast-food restaurant and order and wait for a double cheeseburger and fries, they have time to broil a piece of fish and microwave a potato. Be that as it may, I understand that my seafood lasagna might take too long to prepare after a busy day. But is broiling a chicken breast too time-consuming? Regardless of what I think, the reality is that some will say "yes" and continue to believe that they are "too busy to cook!"

I dedicate the following abridged and simplified two-week *Paty Plan* guide to the sufferers of syndromes one and two. There is little cooking required. The time is limited to grocery shopping, opening a can or two, and occasionally turning on the broiler. Be aware that you will not experience the flavor found in the original plan, but it should satisfy weight-conscious, busy cooking haters.

One final notation: If the following section still does not fit your lifestyle, read the last paragraph found in the chapter "A Final Note."

Two-Week Abridged Paty Plan Menu Suggestions

Sunday

A. Breakfast
   1. One-half cantaloupe

B. Lunch
   1. One can chilled or heated consommé
   2. Seven fat-free saltines
   3. Carrot sticks

C. Dinner
   1. Fat-free turkey slices with two canned lite pear halves
   2. Canned carrots
   3. Canned green beans

Monday

A. Breakfast
   1. Assorted fresh fruit

B. Lunch
   1. Canned artichoke hearts, hearts of palm, cherry tomatoes dipped in fat-free dressing

C. Dinner
   1. One cup canned black beans over one cup instant rice
   2. Ready-to-eat mixed salad greens with fat-free dressing

Tuesday

A. Breakfast
   1. One-half grapefruit

B. Lunch
   1. Canned fat-free soup

C. Dinner
1. One can tuna in water
2. One-half slice pita bread
3. Sliced tomatoes, cucumbers and onions with fat-free dressing

Wednesday

A. Breakfast
1. One-quarter honeydew melon

B. Lunch
1. Ready-to-eat mixed salad greens with raw vegetables and fat-free dressing

C. Dinner
1. Broiled chicken breast *or* fat-free turkey slices with canned cranberry sauce
2. Canned sweet potatoes
3. Canned green beans

Thursday

A. Breakfast
1. One cup fat-free cereal with one-half cup skim milk

B. Lunch
1. One can tuna in water
2. Cut raw vegetables

C. Dinner
1. Canned tomato aspic on lettuce
2. Fat-free cottage cheese
3. Canned asparagus spears

Friday

A. Breakfast
1. One-half grapefruit

B. Lunch
   1. One can chilled or heated consommé
   2. Two large fat-free rice cakes
   3. Carrot sticks

C. Dinner
   1. One cup prepared fat-free tomato pasta sauce over one cup of cooked pasta with fat-free Parmesan cheese
   2. Ready-to-eat mixed salad greens with fat-free dressing

Saturday

A. Breakfast
   1. Sliced melon and berries

B. Lunch
   1. Fat-free ham and cheese pita sandwich with sliced tomatoes

C. Dinner
   1. Three of your favorite canned vegetables

Sunday

A. Breakfast
   1. Crumpet with one tablespoon jam

B. Lunch
   1. Sliced banana and assorted berries

C. Dinner
   1. Broiled fish with lemon or canned fish with no oil
   2. Canned spinach
   3. Sliced cucumbers, tomatoes and onions with fat-free dressing

Monday

A. Breakfast
   1. One-half cantaloupe

B. Lunch
  1. One can chilled or heated consommé
  2. Seven fat-free saltines
  3. Carrots and celery sticks

C. Dinner
  1. Instant grits
  2. Canned corn
  3. Ready-to-eat mixed salad greens with fat-free dressing

Tuesday

A. Breakfast
  1. One-half grapefruit

B. Lunch
  1. Canned fat-free soup

C. Dinner
  1. Three of your favorite canned vegetables (Bake a sweet potato if you can find the time.)

Wednesday

A. Breakfast
  1. Assorted fresh fruit

B. Lunch
  1. Canned artichoke hearts, hearts of palm and cherry tomatoes dipped in fat-free dressing

C. Dinner
  1. Broiled fish with lemon *or* canned fish with no oil
  2. Canned stewed tomatoes
  3. One other canned vegetable

Thursday

A. Breakfast

1. One cup fat-free cereal with one-half cup skim milk

B. Lunch
   1. Assorted fresh fruit

C. Dinner
   1. One cup canned black beans, kidney beans or black-eyed peas over one cup instant rice
   2. Ready-to-eat mixed salad greens with fat-free dressing

Friday

A. Breakfast
   1. One-quarter honeydew melon

B. Lunch
   1. One can tuna in water
   2. Cut raw vegetables

C. Dinner
   1. Broiled chicken breast (or fat-free turkey slices)
   2. Canned sweet potatoes
   3. Canned beets

Saturday

A. Breakfast
   1. One-half grapefruit

B. Lunch
   1. One can tomato aspic
   2. Canned asparagus spears

C. Dinner
   1. Broiled fish with lemon (or canned fish with no oil)
   2. Canned zucchini and tomatoes
   3. Fat-free cottage cheese on a bed of lettuce with sliced yellow and red peppers

The Maintenance Plan

Good news bulletin: You have lost weight!
Sad news bulletin: Keeping your weight off is a lifetime
  commitment.
Great news bulletin: Keeping your weight off is an
  achievable goal!

"Hurrah!" You have just stepped on the scales and your weight loss says it is time to celebrate. It happens to be a summer night and you crave a steak and salad dripping in something other than balsamic vinegar. Go ahead and fire up the charcoal and accompany that porterhouse with a salad tossed with an olive oil vinaigrette. No one deserves it more than the slimmer you. Or perhaps it is a frosty fall day and you want to ladle up a bowl of piping hot beef chili with a piece of French bread smothered in a melting cheddar cheese butter spread. Enjoy your fabulous feast with all my blessings, but with one caveat. These fat-filled indulgences cannot occur on a daily basis. While it may be time to reward your accomplishments, it is also essential that you maintain your new figure.

Maintaining your weight loss is a key ingredient of *The Paty Plan*. The good news is that the maintenance phase is easy and can produce permanent results if you are dedicated. It has been seven years since I ordered my fat-free salad after I left that cocktail buffet untouched. Five years have passed since I reached my desired weight of 125 pounds. I rejoice in the fact that I weigh the same today as I did in December 1995. What is the secret to keeping my weight level? The secret is that I never stray far from *The Paty Plan* list of "do's" and "don'ts." I also live by a three-pound rule. Let me explain.

My husband and I have a fairly busy social schedule with entertaining friends at home or accepting invitations to cocktail and dinner parties. Needless to say, much of this activity is centered around food. At some of these festivities, I throw caution to the wind and satiate myself on forbidden fruits like hot nacho cheese dip or pot roast with potatoes mashed with butter and cream. What happens when I attend several of these events only to discover the needle on the scale inching upward? I never let the weight indicator increase by more than three pounds. How do I do that? I immediately reinstate my ten or less fat gram intake per day methodology. I return to my breakfast and lunch menu suggestion lists and I prepare my beloved turkey breast with a butterless baked potato accompanied with nutritious steamed broccoli for dinner. I normally return to my desired weight within a week following my two-chicken, two-fish, two-vegetable and one-pasta entrée formula. Maintaining your weight loss is that simple.

The recipes in this book are also an integral part of your maintenance program. You should not experience weight gain if you have a low-fat breakfast and lunch and prepare one of my recipes for your main meal.

The last secret to keeping your weight down is exercise. I will repeat once again, eating healthy foods in moderation combined with consistent exercise is the key to a slender figure and hopefully a happier, healthier life.

Be my guest and use a small amount of olive oil when sautéing foods or making salad dressings during the permanent maintenance phase of my plan. Your body, hair and skin require some oils. But do not use a heavy hand or you will see the scales escalate once again.

A Final Note

I have a selfish reason for you to work hard on shedding your excess pounds. I am busy laboring over two new books. *The Dinner Party* and *Cherished Recipes from Northern and Southern Regality* do not promote *The Paty Plan* principles. These cookbooks will present sumptuous recipes for you and your guests to enjoy occasionally at a special dinner party or holiday meal. They will be filled with pre-low-fat-conscious goodies from the days of old. My late mother-in-law's chicken mayonnaise, my grandmother's corn fritters, my mother's duchess potatoes, my melt-in-your-mouth braised lamb shanks. I do not want you to be deprived from time to time of these rich treasures. But it is imperative that you be in a good place physically to moderately indulge in these treats.

If this book is not incentive enough for you to get on the weight loss track, contact me at Festivities, Inc., Post Office Box 12271, Atlanta, Georgia 30355. I will fly, train or bus it to your home for three weeks to ignite your weight loss program. I will plan your strategy, do your grocery shopping and prepare your meals. With this offer there are no excuses left for not getting on the healthy eating bandwagon. Please know it truly would be a pleasure to assist you in realizing your thin dreams.

Appendix

The Paty Plan Recommended Foods

The following is an inventory of low-fat foods to enjoy for a lifetime.

Apples
Applesauce
Apricots
Artichokes
Asparagus
Bananas
Barley
All beans (green, lima, kidney, navy, etc.)
Bean sprouts
Beets
Berries
Most breads
Broccoli
Brussels sprouts
Buttermilk
Cabbage
Angel food cake
Cantaloupe
Carrots
Catsup
Cauliflower
Celery
Cherries
Chicken
Chicory
Clams
Corn
Crab meat
Cranberry sauce
Cream of wheat
Cucumbers
Dates

Egg whites only
Eggplant
Figs
Most fish
Fruit and vegetable juices
Green, red and yellow peppers
Grits
Honey
Honeydew melon
Horseradish
Jams and jelly
Kale
Kiwi
Kumquats
Leeks
Lemons
Limes
Lobster
Mango
Maple syrup
Molasses
Mushrooms
Mussels
Mustard
Nectarines
Oatmeal
Okra
Onions
Oranges
Oysters
Papaya
Parsnips
Dried, non-egg pasta

Peaches
Pears
Peas
Persimmons
Pickles
Pineapple
Plums
Pork tenderloin
Potatoes (white and sweet)
Prunes
Pumpkin
Radishes
Raisins
Rhubarb
Rice

Salad greens
Sauerkraut
Scallops
Shrimp
Summer squash
Winter squash
Strawberries
Tangerines
Tomatoes
Canned tuna fish in water
Turkey
Turnip, collard and beet greens
Turnips
Watermelon
Yams
Zucchini

There is no reason to embellish on the inherent goodness contained in the vegetables found on these pages. Enjoy their natural flavor and benefit from their nutritional properties without adding animal fat to turnip greens or spooning sour cream or grated cheese on your potato.

A reminder to eat the fruits on the list early in the day. Remember also to consume only small amounts of natural sugars like maple syrup and molasses. Sugar supposedly turns to fat.

Stay away from heavily oiled fish like mackerel or blue. Safer bets are flounder, snapper, swordfish, cod and salmon.

Use your common sense. You will only harden arteries, not lose pounds, if you dip your lobster or steamed clams in drawn butter.

The Abridged Paty Plan Weight Loss Guide

Do

1. Consume approximately ten fat grams per day.
2. Remove skin and all visible fat from chicken and fish.
3. Dine on poultry twice a week.
4. Dine on seafood twice a week.
5. Dine on dinners comprised of all vegetables twice a week.
6. Dine on pasta once a week.
7. Eat plenty of vegetables, fruits and lentils.
8. Drink plenty of water.
9. Eat only one serving of bread per day.
10. Exercise.

Do not

1. Eat butter or margarine.
2. Eat foods and salad dressings prepared with oil.
3. Eat mayonnaise.
4. Eat cheese.
5. Eat nuts.
6. Eat egg yolks.
7. Eat olives.
8. Eat avocados.
9. Consume whole milk, half and half, or cream.
10. Eat red meat, organ meat, or ham products, except for pork tenderloin.
11. Eat more than one cup of cooked pasta on pasta nights.

Do Not (continued)

12. Eat bread on the days you are having a cereal or bread product for breakfast.
13. Eat bread on the days you are having a pasta, grits or barley dish for dinner.
14. Eat dessert.

Index

Oven "Fried" Fish, 71
Oven Grilled Vegetable Medley, 81

Parmesan Corn Grits, 64
Parmesan Summer Squash, 58
Poached Fish Rossa with New
    Potatoes, 120

Quick and Easy Italian Dressing, 51

Red Pepper Cole Slaw, 65
Red Pepper Coulis, 52
Rice and Spinach Stuffed Tomatoes,
    104
Roasted Turkey Breast and Stock, 46,
    47

Scallop Pasta Sauce, 62
Scalloped Potatoes, 96
Seafood Florentine, 123
Seafood Lasagna, 78
Seafood Salad, 39
Shrimp and Corn Chowder, 93
Steamed Artichoke, 86
Steamed Mussels with Angel Hair
    Pasta, 55
Summer Salmon and Shrimp, 114

Summer Shrimp and Vegetable
    Salad, 113
Sweet and Sour Glazed Carrots, 83

Tomato and Corn Salsa, 89
Tomato and Yellow Pepper Salsa, 72
Tomato Bruschetta, 94
Tomato Zucchini Soup, 42
Tossed Artichoke Heart and Tomato
    Salad with Creamy Chive
    Vinaigrette, 76
Tossed Marinated Vegetables, 41
Tuna and Pasta Salad, 103
Tuna Pita Bread Sandwich, 37
Turkey, Barley, Vegetable Soup, 117
Turkey Burger, 101
Turkey Enchilada Casserole, 105
Turkey or Chicken Salad Pita Pocket
    Sandwich, 38
Turkey Stroganoff, 85
Turkey Taco Ensalada, 69

Uncreamed Onions, 102

Vegetable Rice Pilaf, 66
Vegetable Stew, 80
Veggie Pita Pizzas, 75

Zippy Italian Lima Beans, 91

About the Author

Katharine Edmonds Paty was raised with Northern roots in Maine and Massachusetts. She received degrees from Bradford College and Lake Forest College. She also studied nineteenth-century French painting at Harvard University and Italian Renaissance art in Florence, Italy. She has resided and worked in the catering business for the past twenty-seven years in Atlanta, Georgia. In 1984 Ms. Paty founded and became president of Festivities, Inc., an event planning company. She is currently working on three new cookbooks including *The Paty Plan—Part Two*.